NATIONAL INSTITUTE SOCIAL SERVICES LIBRARY

Volume 22

THE BOUNDARIES OF CHANGE IN COMMUNITY WORK

THE BOUNDARIES OF CHANGE IN COMMUNITY WORK

Edited by
PAUL HENDERSON, DAVID JONES AND DAVID N. THOMAS

Routledge
Taylor & Francis Group
LONDON AND NEW YORK

First published in 1980 by George Allen & Unwin Ltd.

This edition first published in 2022
by Routledge
2 Park Square, Milton Park, Abingdon, Oxon OX14 4RN

and by Routledge
605 Third Avenue, New York, NY 10158

Routledge is an imprint of the Taylor & Francis Group, an informa business

British Library Cataloguing in Publication Data
A catalogue record for this book is available from the British Library

ISBN: 978-1-03-203381-5 (Set)
ISBN: 978-1-00-321681-0 (Set) (ebk)
ISBN: 978-1-03-204255-8 (Volume 22) (hbk)
ISBN: 978-1-03-204272-5 (Volume 22) (pbk)
ISBN: 978-1-00-319118-6 (Volume 22) (ebk)

DOI: 10.4324/9781003191186

Publisher's Note
The publisher has gone to great lengths to ensure the quality of this reprint but points out that some imperfections in the original copies may be apparent.

Disclaimer
The publisher has made every effort to trace copyright holders and would welcome correspondence from those they have been unable to trace.

The Boundaries of Change in Community Work

Edited by

PAUL HENDERSON
DAVID JONES
DAVID N. THOMAS

London
GEORGE ALLEN & UNWIN
Boston Sydney

First published in 1980

GEORGE ALLEN & UNWIN LTD
40 Museum Street, London WC1A 1LU

British Library Cataloguing in Publication Data

The boundaries of change in community work. –
(National Institute for Social Work. Social
services library; no. 37).
1. Social group work – Great Britain
2. Community development – Great Britain
I. Henderson, Paul II. Jones, David, *b.1942*
III. Thomas, David N IV. Series
361'.941 HV245 79–41603

ISBN 0–04–361038–2
ISBN 0–04–361039–0 Pbk

Typeset in 10 on 11 point Times by Trade Linotype Ltd, Birmingham
and printed in Great Britain
by A. Wheaton & Co. Ltd., Exeter

CONTENTS

ACKNOWLEDGEMENTS

We have enjoyed planning and editing this book; our work was made light by the energy and goodwill of our contributors who responded readily to our suggestions and kept to the timetable that we made for them. As with much of our teaching and writing, we owe most to Jacki Reason and Priscilla Foley. Their advice, support and hard work has ensured so often that we reached the goals we had set for ourselves. Thanks, too, to three of our community work students in 1978/9 who read and commented on parts of the reader – Patrick Bennett, Sarah del Tufo and Chris Warren. We are indebted to Michael Holdsworth of Allen & Unwin who made a crucial contribution to the planning of the book.

We are grateful to Ivor Cutler and Asa Benveniste for permission to use 'Alone', which appeared in *A Flat Man*, Trigram Press, 1977.

NOTES ON CONTRIBUTORS

PETER BALDOCK	Principal Community Worker, Family and Community Services Department, Sheffield
PHIL DORAN	Social Development Officer, Peterborough Development Corporation
CHRIS ELPHICK	Unit Co-ordinator, Community Education Training Unit, Oldham
ROGER ELSE	Principal Planner (Social Policy), Milton Keynes Development Corporation
JALNA HANMER	Lecturer in Community Work, University of Bradford
PAUL HENDERSON	Lecturer in Community Work, National Institute for Social Work
LISA HUBER	Formerly Community Development Officer, Centre for Neighbourhood Development, Belfast
DAVID JONES	Principal, National Institute for Social Work
ISMAIL A. LAMBAT	Community Worker, Longsight/Moss Side Community Project, Manchester; formerly a community worker with Batley Community Development Project
FELICITY MCCARTNEY	Formerly Education Officer, Centre for Neighbourhood Development, Belfast
BRIAN MUNDAY	Senior Lecturer in Social Work, University of Kent
GERALD O'HAGAN	Senior Social Worker, Area 5, Brent Social Services, formerly a community worker with Camden Social Services
GEOFF POULTON	Lecturer in Social Work, Department of Social Work and Social Administration, University of Southampton
HILARY ROSE	Chairperson, Applied Social Studies, Department of Applied Social Studies, University of Bradford

DUDLEY SAVILL	Deputy Head of Social Work Department, Family Housing Association
TERESA SMITH	Lecturer in Applied Social Studies, Department of Applied Social Studies, Oxford
LAURENCE J. TASKER	Lecturer in Applied Social Studies, University of Surrey; formerly at Swansea and Birmingham universities
DAVID N. THOMAS	Lecturer in Community Work, National Institute for Social Work

PREFACE

When we conceived of this book we saw it as an opportunity to take stock of the development of community work in the United Kingdom in the decade since 1968. As we planned the book our intentions somewhat changed in response to ideas that emerged during discussion about what we came to call the 'boundary' nature of community work.

Community work at the boundary developed as the major theme, and our discussion of this theme is presented in the Introduction. We hope that it helps to hold together the chapters in the book. All the contributors were given an early draft of the Introduction, and they were asked to think about their chapters partly, though not wholly, in relation to the boundary theme. Authors in Parts One and Three were also circulated with copies of the case studies of practice.

The introductions to the book and to each of the three parts, together with the concluding commentary, were written by, and are entirely the responsibility of, the editors.

Alone

If
you are mortar
it is
hard
to feel well-disposed
towards
the
two bricks
you are squashed
between
or
even
a sense of
community

IVOR CUTLER

INTRODUCTION: THE BOUNDARIES OF CHANGE IN COMMUNITY WORK

The words and imagery of the poem by Ivor Cutler stimulate sociological interpretations. The bricks seem to represent the different components of which our society is composed – its people, groups, classes and institutions. The stability of the bricks, and the forms they have been used to create, are related to the nature and composition of the foundations. In our society, views of its components, their relations and the ways in which they hold together to create political and sociological forms are rightly influenced by the basic assumptions – one of the foundations – of that society.

There are a number of ways of understanding what mortar represents in this poem. It may be seen as the individuals, groups and interests that are squeezed by the big bricks of society. On the other hand, we could view the mortar as the bonding, integrative elements of society, one of which may be taken to be community work. The integrative nature of community work will be applauded or deplored depending on one's political views and one's appraisal of the basic assumptions upon which one sees society constructed. On the one hand, some might call for more bonding material – even buttresses – to make society more secure, whilst others may choose to press for a falling wall.

Many of the case studies in this book suggest situations in which community workers are caught between various community interests and organisations and yet strive to bond them together (not necessarily without disagreement and conflict) to work on a community issue that transcends particular concerns and boundaries. The bringing and holding together of people in a neighbourhood action group or interdepartmental planning group is, like the mortar in a wall, an essential though sometimes unrecognised job. When we appreciate some fine building, it is not the mortar that our eye naturally lights upon; we ignore its presence, and take for granted the skills and care with which it was prepared and laid. So, too, with community work; it is the organisational forms facilitated by community workers to which we rightly give most of our attention. The most fundamental task for community workers is to bring people together and to help them create and maintain an organisation that will achieve their goals. All other tasks are, in our view, secondary to those of organising people – whether residents or agency staff – into some form of stable and achieving collective.

The task of organising people into a collective has to be achieved by the community worker whilst he or she stands between people and organisations, rather than being of them. Like mortar, their structural position is almost always one of interjacence, carrying out their work on the boundaries of groups and organisations in the community. Community workers have to be with the people, whilst not being of them, and have to develop the additional skill of being able to equilibriate (Halmos, 1978) between the various individuals, groups and organisations that make demands upon them. We wish to use this Introduction to develop the notion of community work as an interjacent activity, lying between other components of society, and in relation to which it has some function. We suggest that ideas and insights about interjacence may be useful for a better understanding of the function and practice of community work, both at a societal and local level.

There is considerable emphasis in the theory and practice of community work on resources, and, in particular, on redistributing them. The resources in question are, on the whole, public resources administered by local and central government departments, other public bodies and voluntary organisations and it is between these bureaucracies and people that community work stands. At the start of Chapter 1, Peter Baldock takes up this theme, and refers to the growth of community action as a response to the functions of modern local government. Community work is, on the one hand, interjacent between organisational interests and, on the other, between individual and collective interests 'out there' in local communities. These individuals and collectivities need not necessarily be of the poor; social action, sometimes involving community workers, has become as much an instrument of the relatively advantaged, as exemplified in campaigns about schooling, motorways, airports, and, as in the case study in Chapter 7 by Roger Else, transport. It is, in effect, an instrument of the powerless, whatever their income and relationship to the means of production; and precisely because of its interjacent nature it is also an instrument that can, and is, employed by the powerful – in this case, local and central government departments.

This perception of community work as lying between people ('clients', 'consumers', 'victims', 'residents') and bureaucracies is not original. It is a perception that occurs in accounts, for example, that point to the isolation and detached position of community workers, and their dual and sometimes multiple lines of accountability to local groups and the agency that employs them. The notion of interjacence is implicit, too, in analyses of community work that suggest its function as a feedback mechanism to corporate and agency management in local authorities. One of the most useful sociological analyses of interjacence is provided by Litwak and Meyer (1966); they write of the antithesis between bureaucracies and community primary groups, and suggest a balance theory of co-ordination between them, one of the links in which may be a detached expert such as a community worker.

We have, then, a picture of community work (at a societal level) and community workers (at a local level) inhabiting the space between local groups and individuals and local and central organisations. In this space, community work and community workers are not static; they move around as they are pushed and pulled by various forces that emanate either from community groups or from bureaucracies. They are impelled, too, by their own internal energy; important policy debates inside community work, or within a group of local workers, will produce a new position in the interjacent space, moving, for example, a group of community workers closer to a chief executive's department or a local trades council. The different members of the bureaucratic environment will differentially push and pull community work and workers; this is a source of anxiety that is revealed in discussions about professionalisation, the 'takeover' of community work by social work and youth work and in fears of co-option and absorption into particular departments. There will always be a concern in community work, if it is to be effective, with 'keeping one's distance' and a fear of being contaminated or sucked in by established professions and agencies. We are not suggesting that the location of interjacence necessarily leads, or should lead, community workers into playing the part of go-between or mediator between community interests. Rather, it is a continually testing drama for community workers both to be in an interjacent location and to resist the temptations of playing the role of link-person where it undermines the authority and competence of community groups. The antipathy in community work to the role of go-between is, perhaps, a justified overreaction to many of the ambiguities inherent in interjacence.

The effects of the push and pull forces on community work and its practitioners will vary with factors such as the cohesiveness and sense of security that is present at any given moment within community work, and with the levels of disorganisation affecting the bureaucracies. The period that followed the establishment of Seebohm departments of social services, for example, may be seen as one in which these departments were able to exert very little cohesive influence on community work. It would be wrong to suppose that the forces or influences that are exerted by bureaucracies or community groups have a uniform effect on community work and community workers. It is our view that the different elements of community work are differentially affected by the push and pull forces in its bureaucratic and community environment; that is, the effect of these forces is to move the 'parts' of community work in different directions from each other. We put parts in quotation marks because we do not want to suggest something that is necessarily tangible.

We want now to consider community work in terms of the tensions that exist between its culture, process of practice, and method of change. We shall take these three for the purposes of introducing the themes and content of this book.

The culture of community work is predominantly other-centred; not only is it in business to serve others, but considerable value is given to the autonomy, power and responsibility of those others, particularly when they are members of community groups. Community work is defined in terms of the struggles of others, and the help and resources that community workers can bring to these struggles; it is difficult to define community work in terms of a corporate professional identity as we can do with social work, teaching and medicine which, unlike community work, expend many resources on their own system's maintenance and development. Its other-centredness is not, on the whole, mitigated by a concern with professional structures and issues, or with identification and affiliation with departments or agencies. The development and expression of itself is not a central feature of community work at the present, though such a concern is becoming apparent in the recent developments connected with training in community work, and referred to in several chapters in this book. Its other-centredness is essentially self-effacing and even subservient, and it is this commitment to others that helps workers to tolerate the isolation, stress, suspicion and lack of support that is often a feature of their work.

The process of the doing of community work, however, is worker-centred; the effectiveness of a worker's transactions with local people depends so much on his or her personality, energy, stamina and skills in the way the worker uses his or her self and resources in a purposeful and disciplined way. The worker has no statutory authority or inducements that facilitate entry and contributions to community groups. If local people or agency staff are turned off him (or her) then there is very little the worker can do, no matter how relevant his or her skills or knowledge, to help a group. The central importance of the worker as an instrument of personal and group change is implicit in the concern in community work with role; in particular, the debate about directiveness and non-directiveness reveals the potency of the benign and adverse effects workers themselves may have on a group.

We do not wish to be misunderstood on this point: we are not suggesting that the worker is or ought to be more important than the group; or that his or her contribution is or ought to be the most central one in achieving the goals that a group has set itself; or that the development of a personal relationship with group members is a more important goal than helping them to organise for effective action. We are rather suggesting that in transactions with a group, or interagency committee, the worker's capacity to be of help to them is primarily a function of the power of person, and through which other bases of influence, such as expertise, are mediated.

The methodological approach to change through community action is we-centred; that is, the values and the instruments of change are essentially those that involve the egalitarianism, fraternity and potency of the collective. The primacy of the collective in community work has three aspects. First, community work is largely concerned with issues and problems in their public or social aspects and is less interested in working with individuals' experience of these problems. It is concerned more with policy than with case, more with collective situations and benefits than with services to particular individuals or families who are in need or disadvantaged. This is not to say, of course, that individuals do not benefit as a result of collective action; in the last resort it is often the individual's estimation of the costs and benefits of community action that may crucially affect the success or failure of collective efforts. Secondly, if the beneficiaries of community action are a larger collective (a street, an estate, a neighbourhood) then, on the whole, benefits are not achieved through individual negotiations, petitioning or protest. The emphasis in community work is on groups of people, whether residents and/or agency staff, taking action in order to secure benefits for a wider population. These first two points suggest that there is in community work a concern with both moral and methodological collectivism.

Thirdly, community work is concerned with participation and with a spirit and methods of working that include people. It thus stresses a collective approach to problem-solving and decision-making about needs, goals, priorities and programmes. In particular, it seeks to enable marginal groups to migrate into 'the acting community' of decisions and decision-makers. This inclusive approach is as much apparent in the case studies that describe work with agencies as in those dealing with neighbourhood groups.

The commitment of service to community and other groups, the worker-centred nature of practice and the collective mode of action in community work combine as the thesis in a dialectic whose antithesis is a fundamental paradox at the heart of the activities of most, but not all, community workers. This antithesis–paradox is that community workers are aligned with the people by identification and principles but they are employed on the whole by local and central state agencies. Community workers stand, as Peter Baldock describes in Chapter 1, 'between the world of welfare professions in which they gain the means to live and the movement for change to which they belong'. They are 'in the welfare state but not of it' but they are also in community groups but seldom, if ever, of them.

One of the syntheses that this dialectic produces is a ragged and changing ideology that acts in its own right as a force that pushes and pulls community work and community workers in the space between local groups and state bureaucracies. The influence of this populist ideology in community work is pervasive and, amongst other things, it serves the purposes of helping workers to believe they are really of and with the people, and of facilitating the division of the world into those who are of and with the people, and those who are with and of the establishment. This division is often present in the debate about whether community work is a social movement or a profession, a matter that is discussed in Chapter 13 by Teresa Smith.

Other effects of this ideology include, for example, the elevation of neighbourhood work and a distaste for social planning and organisational reform and development; a certain romanticisation of the power and abilities of the people; and, as Tasker and Wunnam (1977) have suggested, a radical ethos that produces a sense of moral superiority and self-righteousness in some sections of community work. This constellation of attitudes characterises players in a destructive Bernean game described by Claude Steiner in *The Radical Therapist* (1974) as 'Lefter Than Thou'.

We do not want here to elaborate further on the effects of this populist ideology but rather to suggest that it serves the purpose of helping workers better to bear the paradox we have indicated above, and to disguise the truth about the shifting positions that community work and community workers actually occupy in the space between the people and organisations. The positions shift as community work and community workers are pushed and pulled between their groups and their employers and agency colleagues.

Within each worker there is a constant tension between his or her affiliations and accountability to local groups and those owed, and perhaps felt, towards the agency. Within community work, twists and turns in values, goals and ideas alternatively push and pull community work towards and away from the people; the interest in links with trade unions, for example, may be seen as a force that will emphasise the relationship of workers with local groups rather than with service organisations; the concern about the family as a place of reproduction, and the role of women within it, may also emphasise this relationship. On the other hand, the analysis from the women's movement about the impact of welfare bureaucracies on the family and on women may result in a greater awareness amongst community workers of their organisational affiliations and the opportunities they provide for agency reform and improvement.

Our primary hypothesis is that whilst community work and its practitioners will always be moving around within the space we describe, it will seldom be able or afford to become incorporated either by the people or by the organisations that employ workers. At best, community work and community workers will be anchored to the boundaries of community groups, organisations and professions, and the degrees of externality that are associated with this boundary role may be seen as necessary for the survival and effectiveness of community work. We want now to elaborate on these ideas of interjacence, boundary and externality.

COMMUNITY WORK IN THE INTERJACENCE

Within society, community work occupies a marginal position in relation to major political, economic and social welfare institutions and forces. Community workers tend, on the whole, to work with marginal groups, particularly those left with little in the way of resources, status, power and ambition. Community work stands on the outside of so many important decision-making processes (including those of local groups), yet its function is to help others to move inside decision-making arenas. Community workers may be seen as people who help others to cross boundaries that they themselves invariably remain outside of. This interjacent location of community work is implicitly conveyed in some of the more common role descriptions such as mediator, broker, advocate, facilitator and interpreter. What are the implications for community workers in their practice of being 'outsiders'? We shall briefly examine the relationship of community workers to the local groups with whom they work.

THE COMMUNITY GROUP

The recognition of the boundary nature of community work can be traced time and again in a number of descriptions of community work; these emphasise that it is a process that nearly always involves the application of the skills and knowledge of an external 'expert' or change-agent to indigenous resources in order to undertake action that meets the felt and expressed needs of the local people. Such a conception of community work appears, for example, in Thomason's work, where he writes:

> the basic theorems which underlie the whole process of community work are those which relate to three elements of an influence process:

the agent of influence, the influence process; and the recipient or respondent to influence. In the nature of community work, the community itself functions as an agent in its own (self-) influence, and shares with the external agent in the influence attempt. (1969, p. 24)

The boundary role of the community worker is also implicit in the notion of autonomous community groups that informed the work of the community workers of the London Council of Social Service in the 1960s. Goetschius describes how work with groups was influenced by the four following points of policy:

- advice should only be given on the invitation of the tenants' committee
- a worker could only act for the group at its request
- a worker would offer service to a 'protest' group only if it was willing to discuss its problems
- workers could not join groups as regular members or serve as elected officers. (1971, p. 15)

This policy is, in effect, a series of prescriptions to ensure both the autonomy of the group and the necessarily related externality of the community worker. There is a clear message in many community work texts (see, for example, Jacobs, 1976) that it would be 'out of role' to do anything or to assume a position of membership or leadership that infringed 'group autonomy either by making decisions for the group or by choosing for its members anything that they could reasonably be expected to do, or learn to do, for themselves' (Batten, 1967, p. 13). To be in role in community work is precisely to be external to the group.

The externality of the worker to the community group is viewed in community work theory and practice as both desirable and inevitable. It is desirable because it safeguards the members of a group from the undue influence of the views, values and knowledge of the professional worker; it is in accord with salient values in community work to do with participation and self-determination; and externality is the only status, with its associated roles, that ensures that people learn for themselves how to do things in groups. In addition, the status of externality is essential to foster the long-term independence of the group of the worker, who has to be committed but detached and able objectively to view the activities of the group and its relationships with other systems such as its constituency and the local authority.

Community workers are also outsiders because they are frequently so different from those with whom they work in local groups. With rare exceptions, community workers are outsiders to the groups and their constituencies because of class, education, income, life-style and opportunities. They are professionals come to help others, usually living outside their area, and committed to them for a relatively short period of time. At the outset, community workers are also likely to be more politically aware than the bulk of constituents, or at the very least, more optimistic about the possibilities of collective action and change.

As outsiders, their personal experience of the problems facing local residents is likely to be non-existent or limited, and their analysis of these problems will often be related to events and situations outside of the local community. In his case study in Chapter 6 Gerald O'Hagan refers to the community worker's peripheral perception and experience of the social problems faced by the people resident in a community. The experience of these neighbourhood issues of a professional middle-class community worker who has chosen to live in the community is not the same experience of them that is had by working-class residents, who may not be resident in the area through choice but rather through economic circumstance.

The labels that are used to describe various roles in community work – enabler, catalyst, encourager, educator, and so forth – tend to suggest the contingent nature of the community work intervention, and the status of the worker as someone who is less than a full member of the community and of the groups with whom he or she works. The externality of the community worker will vary with several factors. For example, it will be affected by whether or not he or she is an indigenous worker, and this is explored further in the case study in Chapter 10 by Huber and McCartney; and by the nature of the services or product offered by the worker. The case study in Chapter 5 by Geoff Poulton describes the implications for workers when their product – in this case adult education services – was not seen as usable or desirable by many local people. The case study in Chapter 9 by Ismail A. Lambat is suggestive of the complex way in which the boundary role of the community worker is determined when he or she shares a similar ethnic status to the community members that are being worked with. And Chapter 8 by Dudley Savill on the Association of London Housing Estates indicates that many of the ambiguities and tensions of interjacence are present even when the community worker is employed by community residents.

It is, of course, unsatisfactory to draw attention only to the 'outsideness' of the community work role. The situation for the worker, and for community work within society at large, is more complex. Community workers have also to build up working relationships with community group members; in order to be effective they have to become accepted, trusted and valued as contributing something to the work of the group. They have to get close to people and issues, being seen as committed to the goals and interests of the group. Being accepted as an 'insider', albeit a temporary one, is undoubtedly a condition for effectiveness in community work. This suggests that one of the skill areas in community work is that of maintaining a creative tension between the 'in' and 'out' aspects of one's role, and being able to manage the ambivalence both of the role and of the feelings that it creates in oneself and group members. This point is further discussed in Chapter 11 by Brian Munday.

Much the same may be said of workers' relationships to their employing agency. Being effective in achieving change within the agency may equally depend on workers being accepted and valued as members of the group, even though this perception of the workers by others (and by themselves) will necessarily co-exist with their reality as marginal or boundary persons in the agency.

The externality of the community worker may also be an important requirement for effective work in the field of interorganisational relationships. The success of workers in facilitating joint planning and co-ordination between agencies may depend on their being seen as the 'disinterested middle-man', not associated with the particular interests of any one of the agencies involved in the co-ordinating process. The capacity of community workers to bring together different departments or community interests is exemplified in Chapters 6, 7 and 10 by O'Hagan, Else, and Huber and McCartney. There is an episode in the chapter by Else in which he describes his position in a meeting between the development corporation and a transport users' group. The reality and delicacy of the worker's interjacent position is powerfully conveyed in Else's description of the meeting. There is a strong sense in all three chapters that the worker's abilities successfully to bring people together and to provide essential back-up tasks is a function not only of the worker's 'time, effort, energy, thought and imagination' but also of his or her interjacence and externality of role.

The boundary nature of the community work role may be seen as a purely developmental phenomenon, associated with the relative newness of community work in this country. Our view, however, is that the role of community work in acting upon, and moving between, the boundaries of organisations, may also be understood as a structural factor that is a function of the very nature of community work itself. It may be more appropriate to realise that the kind of contribution that community workers are able to make to community groups and their service agencies is in important ways dependent on the preservation of their 'outsideness'. Incorporation into any of the systems that are worked with may endanger the integrity and the vitality of the community work role by diluting the critical and supportive faculties that community workers bring to bear on the situations of community groups and community organisations. Co-option is justifiably a suspect word amongst community workers; the emotions it arouses epitomise a fear of all states of incorporation. The community work task has to remain external to community groups and service organisations because it is an operating condition that supports the survival and distinctive contribution of community work. The community worker is a marginal person and an intermediary precisely because that is what he or she is and what he or she has to be in order to be an effective change-agent within a pluralist community environment of competing interests.

THIS BOOK

We hope that some of the ideas that we have tentatively raised in this Introduction – those of interjacence, boundary and externality, for example – are of sufficient interest not only to encourage the reader to explore them further in relation to community work, but also to provide a broad theme for the book that will hold together and provide continuities between the different chapters. Such continuities will sometimes be explicit where an author uses, for instance, the notion of boundary-ness to highlight a particular point of interest in his or her work. More often, perhaps, these continuities in the book will be there waiting to be discovered by the reader who is willing to think about some of the key concepts discussed in this Introduction and bring them to bear on what he or she finds in the chapters in the book. We suggest that the notions of interjacence, boundary and externality provide a potentially productive set of analytic tools for thinking about community work. We have only been able to signpost in this Introduction some of the possible areas of discussion and insight that they make possible; a map has been provided for an intellectual journey that others can undertake.

The hub of the book is a selection of case studies which describe a number of settings, geographical locations and groups with and in which community workers work. No selection of studies of practice will win universal acclaim; there are many examples of practice that we have not been able to include because of considerations of space. It would be foolish for us to claim that these case studies, or any other selection, were typical or representative of community work in Britain. We trust, however, that they are suggestive of the variety of activities that comprise community work in Britain and that they provide material for the reader to reflect upon the ideas of interjacence, boundary and externality.

Part One of the book provides an opportunity to understand the import of these ideas in relation to the historical origins of community work, and in the diversity of values and theories that inform community work practice. One of the characteristics of an interjacent activity such as community work is that its origins and points of growth will be closely connected to, and confused by, the origins and development of other activities, movements, individuals and organisations with which it is related. Another way of making this point is to reflect that in the making of community work we may discern important changes in the policies and practices of other organisations and professions. In particular, Chapter 1 by Peter Baldock and Chapter 11 by Brian Munday in Part Three, suggest how closely linked is the development of community work values and practice to a sense of dissatisfaction in and with many of the organisations and professions with which community work has been associated. Peter Baldock's chapter can be seen, within the confines of this book, as a precursor of a fuller historical treatment, as laying the basis of further work to be done. It adds, too, to the historical analysis already begun by Baldock in an article in the *Community Development Journal* (1977).

Nick Derricourt has remarked that 'there is next to no community work theory *per se* but it is important that the theoretical contributions of other disciplines should be drawn together' (1977, p. 143). It may be the fate of an interjacent activity such as community work that it needs to beg, borrow and steal its theoretical structures. Just as workers operate in their day-to-day work in the space between organisations and groups, so, too, do they seem to move between different disciplines (social work, adult education, political theory, the social sciences), picking and choosing relevant bits of theory and research to structure their own activities.

The areas of knowledge and skill expected of community workers by residents and agency staff have been indicated by Derricourt, and in publications from the Central Council for Education and Training in Social Work and the Association of Community Workers; the elements in their practice about which workers need some understanding have been summarised by Peter Leonard (1977) as the community or neighbourhood in which the worker is employed; the local organisational and political context; the wider structural variables; and the community work intervention process itself. From these four elements alone we can conceive of the variety of explanations or theories that are available to workers. In understanding these elements, community workers will find themselves on the boundary between, on the one hand, political, economic or environmental explanations and, on the other, of explanations that give more emphasis to individual and group phenomena. That is, workers need recourse to theories and ideas that provide some structural understanding of local issues, but they also need a framework for understanding the actors, including themselves, in the local situation. This is one of the themes developed in Chapter 3 by Jalna Hanmer and Hilary Rose who speak of the need to integrate personal experience with a conceptual understanding of the world.

In a sense, community workers find themselves on the boundaries of the various disciplines that comprise the political and social sciences, seeking explanations of the individual, group, community and structural dimensions of community affairs. Of course, workers may give more weight to some kinds of explanations than others, and this may be most apparent in their writings and public statements; in practice, however, each worker's effectiveness will depend, amongst other factors, on the ease with which they can negotiate the boundaries of different kinds of explanations and theoretical frameworks, some of which are suggested by Laurence Tasker in Chapter 2, and in Chapter 3 by Hanmer and Rose.

In the paper (1977) referred to earlier, Peter Leonard makes the distinction between descriptive, explanatory theory and prescriptive theory. Here Leonard highlights one of the most painful intellectual boundaries on which community workers stand, because our explanations of the causes and persistence of local or neighbourhood disadvantage often do not entail or even suggest what the prescription or strategy for action is at the local level. There are two related issues about theory that overlay this one. First, there is the continuing distaste in community work of theory, partly because of suspicions of its distancing power, and partly because of a scepticism that recognises the socially constructed nature of theory and ideas. Secondly, whatever the attitudes of workers to theory they must often find themselves on the boundary between thought and emotion. The complexity of the causes and persistence of disadvantage demands critical analysis and clear thought; yet the contact of the worker with deprivation, powerlessness, suffering and stigma evince an emotional response, engendering identification, commitment and involvement. Both analysis and effect are necessary to the worker, though they are not necessarily compatible, the one sometimes inhibiting the other. The boundary between analysis and effect is one of the most crucial to be negotiated.

It is not helpful to view the varied and eclectic theoretical (and value) base as a purely opportunistic factor; it is usefully seen as reflecting the pressures and practical requirements of an external occupational role. Community work may need to resist incorporation into any particular value or knowledge system as much as it needs to resist incorporation into organisational systems. Perhaps the effectiveness and personal survival of workers operating on the margins of, and in the space between, a variety of groups and organisations may depend on their being able to draw upon a wide range of explanatory, prescriptive and evaluative frameworks. Normative and theoretical narrowness or rigidity may imperil workers' effectiveness and, indeed, push them towards incorporation within a community or organisational system that allows them comfortably to work within a narrow band of effectiveness. This may occur where that system operates from a similarly constrained value and knowledge base or where the work that it presents is always such that it allows the worker to be effective simply because it is amenable to the particular perspectives and approach of the worker. Move away from that system and that work, and the worker becomes a fish out of water.

The ideas of interjacence and boundary serve, too, to sharpen our awareness about the status and content of values and ideology in community work and amongst its practitioners. It would be misleading to think that community work in Britain was inspired by one particular set of values; Jerry Smith (1978) has helpfully written about four ideologies: the Conservative, the Liberal/Democrat, the Libertarian and the Marxist.

As with the historical origins of community work, it is difficult because of the realities of interjacence to discern in the values and ideologies of community workers anything that may be said to be particular to community work. Rather, it seems to us that the primary value sets in community work are closely linked to, and often are derivable from, prevailing values in other professions, organisations and movements. More significantly, the reality of interjacence and the need for workers to move between a variety of organisational and group interests suggest to us the possibility that the effectiveness of community workers depends in part on these other interests not perceiving community work to be dominated by any particular value commitment. It may be that the emergence of a definable and widely accepted value position (whether defined morally or politically) in community work would work adversely against the ability of community workers to equilibriate between community interests, and thus to carry out their fundamental task of helping people in communities and agencies to organise. This is not to suggest that community workers are or ought to be bland or neutral or uncommitted on the important social issues of the community or society. This would be impossible for many and undesirable for all as Chris Elphick suggests at the end of his case study in Chapter 4.

Our view is that community work as a system, or any subsystem of it, must strive to maintain variety and reasoned uncertainty in its set of values. Homogeneity in values might be achieved only at the cost of operational effectiveness; dogmatism and closed value boundaries may jeopardise the ability to organise. This calls for a great deal of skill and imposes considerable strain within community work. What is being asked for is that an occupation whose practitioners are intimately concerned with the effects on communities of major social, political and economic forces refrains from developing a uniform occupational ideological 'position' that is applied doctrinally to these issues. This does not entail having no views about these issues, and nor does it entail the diminution of ideology as a force in community work, or the presence of ideology as a factor in a worker's decisions about practice.

Community work is blessed by an in-built counter against the emergence of a more or less unified occupational ideology; this is the diversity to be found in the values, interests and styles of its practitioners. Interjacence fortunately provides the opportunity for a wide variety of people to enter community work, and this fact sustains the pluralism and openness necessary in the occupation for its workers to be allowed to equilibriate between community interests in an attempt to oiganise them for collective action.

The diversity of practitioners in community work is related to two other issues, both of which are important for the development of interjacent and boundary roles. The first is the great variety of jobs that may be lumped within the practice of community work; and the second is the extent to which community work remains an open and non-exclusive occupation, a factor which helps to produce the personnel to undertake the range of jobs community work is asked to embrace. We want to discuss only the first of these issues, and to suggest that it is inevitable and perhaps desirable that because of interjacence, community work as an occupation is asked to take on a variety of tasks, and to accept a number of interpretations of its work and role.

No one definition or approach in community work is on *a priori* grounds necessarily more worthwhile or relevant than any other. The value and relėvance of a particular approach or practice (the choice, for example, between community care and community action) must be decided upon by the local factors – largely the views and felt needs of residents – that each practitioner must take into account in making decisions about the nature and direction of his or her work. More importantly, it may be the case that in order for its practitioners to operate effectively within interjacent and boundary roles it is necessary for community work as an occupation, first, to resist too narrow or dogmatic definition of the tasks of community work lest such a definition closes off the freedom for workers to undertake their organising tasks and, secondly, to allow community and agency needs to define the nature of the community work tasks (and the parameters of community work as an occupation).

This is not to say, however, that individual workers must remain unclear about what they are to do, or must necessarily accept the role of dustbin and carry out all the tasks that other people in their agency are loth or unskilled to take on. To argue that community work as an occupation must remain catholic in the tasks and roles it is prepared to consider within its boundaries does not entail that individual workers, or their employers, should be indiscriminating in their choice of work. Rather, the inclusiveness of the occupation allows its practitioners the opportunity and professional legitimation to work on one set of local issues as against many others that were open to them.

Individual community workers must be sensitive to whether or not covertness or openness about their values and ideology will help, in each situation they find themselves in, in the task of holding the interjacent ground in order to organise. As Van Hoffman has wisely cautioned, if you are vegetarian, do not make a fad or issue about it in the community because you may find that you need the support of the neighbourhood butchers. To be passionate in one's feelings about issues, and yet to be quiet and modest, where necessary, in the expression of them, is a requirement of sustained and successful work on the boundaries of community interests.

An important assumption here is that community workers must be free to move in the interjacence and to organise, and that the way in which community work's and the individual community worker's values are perceived by others will enhance or diminish this freedom of movement. The presence of freedom on manoeuvre is partly a function of structure, and in particular the nature of the worker's employment situation, and partly dependent on the worker's own skills and creativity. It is, too, greatly dependent on what is allowed to him or her by the various community interests between whom the worker lies. It is thus important to try to understand more about community work as an occupation and/or profession, and about its sponsorship by and permeation of local and national organisations. This is the task we have set ourselves in Part Three of the book.

In order to work successfully in the interjacence, community work and its practitioners must have relatively open boundaries. This fact has a number of consequences for community work, some of which are discussed in Part Three. The identity and occupational development of community work will be determined not only by what its practitioners and organising bodies decide, but also by the organisations and groups with whom it interacts. The fact of interjacence necessarily introduces a transactive element into the evolution of community work as an occupation, and some of the forces in this evolution are indicated in Chapter 13 by Teresa Smith. But, as Brian Munday documents in Chapter 11, the fact of transaction leads to the permeation of other occupations and professions by community work, and the 'slippage' of the language, ideas and priorities of community work into these other spheres.

The issue of sponsorship of community work has received considerable attention in the American literature on community work, but until recently it has been difficult to find in British literature appraisals, particularly based on experience and research, of matters to do with management and supervision. The question of who employs the community worker is clearly a crucial one in relation to interjacence, and we have already discussed some of the issues earlier in this Introduction. Chapter 12 by Phil Doran takes this discussion further, and provides material to help us think about the varying opportunities and constraints present in different employment situations that affect the ability of practitioners to move about in the interjacence.

Doran's chapter also provides a link between the first and last parts of the book because he discusses the effect of the values, theories and training of workers on their employment situation. The nature of the relationship of the worker with the employing agency may be seen as the product of what the worker brings across the boundaries of the agency and some salient features of the agency structure such as funding and decision-making processes.

The ambivalence of community workers to their employing agencies, the lack of understanding of their role and activities amongst their colleagues, their critical appraisal of their agency's services and operating procedures, and differences in their values and training, all help to ensure that community workers will tend to remain on or near the boundaries of the agencies that employ them. The authors of one study have suggested that this is particularly the case with community workers employed in social services departments:

> many community workers are only marginal members of their area group . . . [they] seem to be members of the department only insofar as it pays their salaries, provides minimal resources such as a desk and telephone, and gives some general mandate for their work. We believe that the neighbourhood interventions of many community workers are 'grafted' onto the social services department and that their area group is, in effect, a 'host' system for a range of goals, values, strategies and activities that remain unintegrated within those of the department. (Thomas and Warburton, 1977, p. 25)

The boundary position of the worker will often be consolidated in agencies by other facts: he or she is likely to be the only community worker in the agency and will often not be a member of any subteam in the agency. In addition, community workers can be expected to have different work patterns from their colleagues and be less able and willing to produce immediate or tangible 'results' from their work. The activities of the worker are unlikely, too, to be within the mainstream of the agency's business; indeed, many agencies look to community workers to provide a criticism of, and alternatives to, the traditional or routinised responses of the agency to individual and social needs.

Community work has developed in this country largely on the boundaries of existing organisations, with community workers contributing to the work of a variety of different agencies but remaining unintegrated within their overall policies and goals (and indeed, wanting to change them). At the same time, community work has only slowly and with some reluctance set about building its own professional and occupational base. Community work faces an interesting paradox: on the one hand, as a relatively new development its practitioners must face the task of building up community work as a distinctive method of intervention with well-articulated proposals about values, theories, training and expertise. On the other hand, energies and resources are diverted away from this task partly because it is the nature of community work to contribute to the development and identity of other professions and organisations.

Thus we seem to find community work servicing a whole range of organisations, and influencing many aspects of British political, social and administrative life, but at the expense of its own organsational and theoretical development. It is the aspects of this paradox that are also explored by the contributors to Part Three of the book. This section highlights some of the forces to which community work and its practitioners are exposed as a result of the different, and perhaps often irreconcilable, demands made on them by the organisations with and for whom they work, their professional peer group of community workers, and their own needs for professional autonomy and freedom from organisational and political constraints.

REFERENCES

Baldock, P. (1977). 'Why community action? The historical origins of the radical trend in community work', *Community Development Journal* vol. 12, no. 2 (April).

Batten, T. R. (1967) *The Non-Directive Approach in Group and Community Work* (London: OUP).

Derricourt, N. J. (1977). 'Linking learning to experience in community work training', in C. Briscoe and D. N. Thomas (eds), *Community Work: Learning and Supervision* (London: Allen & Unwin).

Goetschius, G. (1971). *Working with Community Groups* (London: Routledge).

Jacobs, S. (1976). *The Right to a Decent House* (London: Routledge).

Halmos, P. (1978). *The Personal and the Political: Social Work and Political Action:* (London Hutchinson).

Leonard, P. (1977). 'The contribution of the social sciences: ideology and explanation', in C. Briscoe and D. N. Thomas (eds), *Community Work: Learning and Supervision* (London: Allen & Unwin).

Litwak, E. and Meyer, H. J. (1966). 'A balance theory of co-ordination between bureaucratic organisations and community primary groups', *Administrative Science Quarterly*, vol. 11.

Smith, J. (1978). 'Possibilities for a socialist community work practice', in *Towards a Definition of Community Work* (London: ACW).

Steiner, C. (1974). 'Radical psychiatry and movement groups', in *The Radical Therapist* (ed.), The Radical Therapist Collective (Harmondsworth: Penguin).

Tasker, L. and Wunnam, A. (1977). 'The ethos of radical social workers and community workers', *Social Work Today*, vol. 8, no. 23 (15 March).

Thomas, D. N. and Warburton, R. W. (1977). 'Staff development in community work in social services departments', in C. Briscoe and D. N. Thomas (eds), *Community Work: Learning and Supervision* (London: Allen & Unwin). The report of the case study is *Community Workers in a Social Services Department: A Case Study* (London: NISW/PSSC, 1977).

Thomason, G. (1969) *The Professional Approach to Community Work* (London: Sands).

PART ONE

THE CONTEXT OF COMMUNITY WORK PRACTICE

INTRODUCTION

Community work has a history, but one that needs to be written. The complex skeins which surround its origins are only beginning to be untangled, and there are still only occasional glimpses to be had of the breadth and richness which historical study of community work in Britain must yield; for example, in Chapter 3 Jalna Hanmer and Hilary Rose reflect on how far the shifts in approaches to community development can be matched by the movements of particular individuals. There is scope for biography as well as autobiography. Furthermore, the historian has to explore both the day-to-day functioning of community projects with their mass of detail, and the relationship of community work to major issues and themes in society at any one time. Understanding the origins and development of community work requires, in this sense, a combination of sympathetic insight into what happens in community work practice with a rigorous approach to policy analysis.

Concern with community work's history is far from being of merely academic interest. At the level of practice, when community workers apply their knowledge and skills, an understanding of the history of organising for collective action outside the workplace has been haphazard at best. This matters, because it means that not as much is learnt from previous projects and experiments as might be. In addition, an awareness and understanding of past traditions and practices represents an essential analytic tool for community workers and one which they have tended to neglect. An historical awareness is perhaps a necessary attribute of an emerging occupation.

In using the word 'context' for this part of the book we seek to imply the idea of relating parts to one another, parts which are hard to define precisely and which can stimulate varied interpretations. It is one way of seeking to understand the development of community work practice. The three chapters can be seen as contributing to building up a context of community work, thereby adding to the conceptual base which practitioners can draw upon. Readers will note, for example, how all the authors emphasise the significance of the women's movement for community work.

In Chapter I, Peter Baldock, while drawing attention to its diverse and fascinating origins, reminds us that 'community work is still at the end of its beginning', despite the expansion of employment in community work over the last twelve years. He also suggests that it corresponds most closely to a professionalism which is a compromise between social movement and state bureaucracy, and it is interesting to compare his analysis of this topic with that of Teresa Smith in Part Three, Chapter 13. His contention that the development of community work can be seen essentially as a response to change is argued by reference to key turning points in the growth of community work. The chapter provides an historical map to enable readers to find their bearings.

The other two chapters can be seen as filling in particular areas of this map in more detail, while sharing with Baldock a commitment to fostering a more comprehensive historical analysis of community work. In Chapter 2, Laurence Tasker elucidates four categories of theories which relate to current ideas in community work practice. His identification of contextual theory and practice as the probable priority area for theorising in community work implies 'a dynamically oriented sociology', monitoring, and the more systematic collection of data. This, bearing in mind the wide range of projects which provide bases for community work, will demand more research resources as well as a firmer commitment to theory itself.

The identification by Jalna Hanmer and Hilary Rose in Chapter 3 of 'a more critical and self-sceptical mould' within community work is one stimulus to the interest 'both in present theoretical issues and also in a re-examination of the roots of community work itself'. Their chapter begins by drawing attention to the colonial inheritance of community work in Britain before discussing three competing paradigms of social work: the consensual, and pluralist and structural versions of conflict theory. Alongside a continuing enthusiasm for community work practice there has evolved 'a recognition that we have to make sense of practice in theoretical terms'. Jalna Hanmer and Hilary Rose offer such an understanding by analysis of the feminist movement.

Laurence Tasker's first category of theory – social policy – provides a further clue to the common thrust of the chapters in this part, for it is concerned with where 'community work fits in an overall strategy of services to and control of society'. It is the nature of the relationship between the parts which are relevant to the development of community work practice that constitute the context we are searching for. The historical map provided by Baldock enables the other authors not only to focus on selected aspects of it but also to put forward important ideas about community work theory, values and ideologies. It is to be noted that all the authors are concerned to understand this context by examining it from the bottom, that is from the experience of the practitioners and the recipients of community work. History or theory which drifts away from that starting point will fail to provide either an accurate or useful contextual framework for practice.

Chapter 1

THE ORIGINS OF COMMUNITY WORK IN THE UNITED KINGDOM

Peter Baldock

In the minds of many, community work sprang into being fully grown like Athene from the head of Zeus. All of a sudden there was a lot of it about. The impression is deceptive. Community work has a history that stretches back to the 1880s and has its roots in developments that have a still longer history.

It is, of course, possible to exaggerate the antiquity of community work. As a reasonably well-defined occupation it is a very recent arrival on the scene. Community action, with which paid community work has a rather complicated relationship, is also something comparatively new. When Hebditch (1976) attempts to trace its origins back to Ket's rebellion in the sixteenth century he is making a contribution to mythology rather than history. Community action – in the sense intended by, for example, the publishers of the magazine of that name – is a response to the growth of local government, so that one has to be cautious in describing even nineteenth-century movements as providing its origins.

As an example of working-class collective action, community action obviously has some features in common with, for example, the co-operative movement of the Rochdale Pioneers. But that nineteenth-century movement represented a step away from political and industrial agitation as Chartism began to fail, while community action represents a step into it rendered necessary by the functions of modern local government. The Pioneers thus had more in common with the various thrift societies of their own time than with modern community action. Their chronicler Holyoake (1893, pp. 11–13) betrays a positive embarrassment in recording the last lingering echoes of revolutionary fervour in the early days of the Pioneers. It is, besides, difficult to trace any connection between the direct heirs of the Pioneers and the activists in community action. Elsewhere there has been similarity of response in similar circumstances without their being an organic link. It is doubtful whether the rent-striking women in Govan in 1915 were aware of the similarity of their action to that of the women bread rioters during the Napoleonic Wars. Even over shorter periods of history there can be similarity without direct connection. There was little, for example, between the squatters of the 1960s and those of the 1940s.

If community action is a recent development, community work as an occupation is even more so. One can trace the social origins of modern community work back nearly two centuries. By contrast, the particular notions in which community work had its origins are little more than ninety years old. And it is only recently that a distinct occupation has emerged.

ASPECTS OF MODERN SOCIETY

The triumph of the capitalist mode of production in the nineteenth century brought with it a phenomenal material growth that half intoxicated and half terrified the class that benefited most from what was being achieved. The massive developments of the cities occurred too rapidly for any significant planning to be possible. But cholera and riots demonstrated the foolishness of allowing unorganised expansion.

In the first half of the century it was precisely those who were most implacable in the suppression of working-class discontent who were often the most active in reform. One could cite the industrialists who built model villages for their own workforces – Salt, Price and Ashworth – or Chadwick, creator of the Poor Law 'bastilles', but also of modern urban management, or Shaftesbury, profoundly conservative in many of his views, but also the leading pioneer in social legislation. The occasional deviant from this pattern, notably Robert Owen, is important in the history of socialist thought, but for that very reason a departure from the general pattern of his own time.

In a period of rapid economic change the interests of conservatism itself made reform necessary. In some cases, reform could be positively against the interests of the poor, as Nevitt (1966, pp. 77–80) demonstrates. Even among those with a more humane outlook – people like Octavia Hill, Ebenezer Howard or Patrick Geddes who were the pioneers of such professions as social work, housing management and town planning – the dominant attitude was one of benevolent authoritarianism. It was because of the needs of the dominant classes that the political history of the nineteenth century became one of institutional reform and development – the creation of new political structures, the development of the notion of public health, the invention of town planning and social work, the political concern with housing provision and (last of all, as the inadequacies of an aggressive ideology of individual self-reliance became glaringly obvious) the beginnings of the welfare state.

There was, of course, an alternative perspective to that of the dominant classes and their agents – the perspective of those who primarily suffered from the violence of change and the inhumanity of power. But that perspective was never half so well articulated. An instinct or even habit of rebellion existed. But the language in which it developed had to be borrowed from the dominant class, and this inevitably detracted from the success of that articulation.

The question of housing and town planning is typical in this respect. While the intelligent middle class were very much concerned in the last century with the question of working-class housing, a parallel concern rarely found expression in the labour movement. When Engels in the 1870s attacked Mülberger's plan for providing mortgage facilities for workers, he accurately pointed out the conservative implications of the proposed reform, but totally failed to show any appreciation himself of the issues involved, seeing housing as a simple matter of the supply of something whose actual nature was to be taken for granted (Engels, 1956). Engels's attitude was as typical as it was influential. In the earlier part of the century, there were initiatives under Owenite influence in some areas, such as those that led to the creation of Walkley as the 'working-man's West End' in Sheffield. Towards the end of the century there were occasional campaigns such as that of the Tenants' Defence League in Wolverhampton. But, on the whole, the labour movement's interest in housing as an issue followed on from Conservative and Liberal reforms and was largely a response to them. Even the rent control achieved by the Great Glasgow Rent Strike of 1915 was already well in the minds of the government as a counter-inflation measure, and even after the war one can still find Labour spokesmen who were dubious about radical housing reform, men as influential as J. H. Thompson (1920, p. 74). Since then both the Labour Party and other groups further to the left have been characterised in their housing policy, on the whole, by a concern to provide, combined with a relative unenthusiasm about owner-occupation, but not by any sophisticated understanding of the city as such.

Nevertheless, the increasing importance of housing policy in the lives of working-class families was one of the reasons why, outside the trade union struggle, the primary feature of the Labour movement from the end of the nineteenth century to the close of the Second World War was the achievement of power in local government through local Labour Parties that had been built up on a base of local industrial solidarity – a kind of parochialism that contrasted significantly with Marx's concept of the world historical role of the proletariat.

Clay Cross was, perhaps, the last instance of the achievement of local power by militant labourism in this kind of way.

It is not only that local government reorganisation has removed many of the opportunities for this sort of development. Solidarity based on common residence and occupation is in decline and within the socialist movement is now being complemented, if not replaced, by newer forms of solidarity based on common consciousness of oppression as a sex, or race, or generation, or stigmatised minority, or a group at the receiving end of the ambiguous benefits of some agency of the welfare state. The women's movement is the most crucial of these developments and is particularly crucial to community work, as Mayo's recent book (1977) has gone some way to demonstrating.

One of the ways in which the dominance of middle-class ideology manifested itself in the nineteenth century Labour movement was in the widespread acceptance of patriarchal ideas on the role of women. As the first really large affluent class in human history, the Victorian middle class developed a style of family life that differed from much that had gone before. The family became less important as a unit of production, more so as a unit of consumption. It provided the private sphere in which compensations were sought for the frustrations of the world of work. Families became smaller and more intimate. The working class followed in the footsteps of its betters. But, once affluence was more or less achieved, a re-examination of the nature of the family became possible. If personal gratification was the aim, then the patriarchal system was an irrelevance. Both sexual 'permissiveness' and militant feminism followed. There was, of course, a degree of ambivalence about all this. The family not only represented the sphere of freedom, it also performed the vital function of educating its members to accept social norms. Other mechanisms were becoming available (such as universal schooling and the mass media), but the importance of the family could not be ignored. Thus both permissiveness and feminism were controversial and the controversy expressed itself in tensions in actual families as well as in debates in the columns of newspapers.

Within twentieth-century feminism there have been two main currents. One has seen women's liberation as the key issue for women. Another has seen it as an integral part of the struggle of all men and women for freedom and has emphasised the part that the oppression of women plays in the maintenance of capitalist society. As articulated theories both are likely to be found mainly among educated women. But they correspond approximately to two rather different generators of feminist revolt. Many of those in the actual women's liberation movement are among the more affluent and better educated whose expectations for themselves contrast with the standard roles of wife and mother. On the other hand, many less affluent women are driven to rebellion because society does not allow them the means to play the roles expected of them – means such as decent housing. The two forms of women's rebellion are often in little more than fluctuating contact with one another, although there have been times and places where effective alliances have been made and lessons learnt. Perhaps the most valuable of these experiences (because there has been some kind of institutional infrastructure to ensure continuity and development) has been in the refuges for battered women organised by Women's Aid groups.

In all that has been said so far – on Victorian middle-class movements for social reform, on the hesitant way in which the Labour movement has taken up issues outside industry and government, and on newer forms of socialism that emphasise the equal importance of the so-called 'private' sphere – the emphasis has been on change. The Victorians, who sometimes have a reputation for being staid and unimaginative, were amazingly inventive. 'What creed, what doctrine, what institution was there among them which was not at some time or other debated or assailed?' asks Young and says 'I can think of two only: Representative Institutions and the Family' (1953, p. 150). Now, of course, even those are in doubt – the latter as a result of the changes in family life already indicated, the first with a good deal of loose, but still significant, talk in the late 70s of the 'ungovernability' of Britain. Change on the scale that our society has experienced in the last two hundred years must bring anxiety as well as exhilaration. The anxiety arises less from a fear of specific evils, than from the incomprehensible, unpredictable nature of social existence today. It is possible to overdramatise, but not to overemphasise this prevailing note of uncertainty. As another finger is put in another hole, the dyke starts leaking somewhere else. So far there has been no great shortage of fingers, though some have taken longer to arrive than others. But the flurry of activity is itself a cause of disquiet.

A crucial part in this has been played by the new black minorities in Britain. It is not only the fact that 'immigrants' provide a convenient scapegoat for the shortage of houses or jobs that explains the spread of racism. Their arrival coincided with the fall of the British Empire and served as a reminder that the world role in which Britain once seemed secure had been lost. And, of course, simply by living in their own way they contribute to a general cognitive dissonance. The manipulative Jew was always a mere figment of racist imagination. As the third world on the doorstep, the 'immigrant' really does represent some kind of threat to the narrower prejudices of British society.

Community work has been one of the responses to the situation of complication and uncertainty that has been sketched so far. At times it has been a conservative response, at other times more radical. Indeed, the major feature of the history of community work in the UK has been the way in which an essentially conservative movement at the moment of its partial acceptance by the state took an oddly radical turn. But both conservative and radical community workers have been responding to essentially the same conditions.

THE DEVELOPMENT OF THE IDEA OF COMMUNITY WORK

As a response to the condition of uncertainty, community work only became conceivable when that condition reached a certain pitch. An important element in the determination of that pitch was probably the erosion of religious faith in the middle of the last century. To the extent that community work is an attempt to respond to moral confusion, it has taken on something of the role of the churches. Indeed, the man who has the best claim to be considered the first British community worker was a parish priest in the Church of England.

Samuel Barnett is one of the most important and currently underrated figures in the history of social welfare. A case has been recently made that his view of the degradation of the poor as a consequence rather than the cause of their poverty was an ideological breakthrough in Victorian social-work circles (Leat, 1975). His radicalism in this respect can be exaggerated. 'Classes must exist', he said, and his 'set determination to regard all men as brothers' had much in common with C. S. Loch's view of the Charity Organisation Society (COS) as a 'Great Companionship of Charity, West with East, rich with poor, the elder with the younger generation' (Loch, 1885). Barnett's policies on the Whitechapel Board of Guardians were in accordance with the strictest requirements of the dogmaticians of the COS, leading, indeed, to riots. Like others, he did drift away from those principles to some extent, enough at any rate to be the victim of a quite vitriolic personal attack by Loch at a COS council meeting in 1905. But his real inventiveness did not lie in the fact that he followed a general trend towards Fabian socialism. It lay in the way that he devised a new type of agency – the settlement – that represented, like the COS itself, an attempt to put certain principles into methodical practice.

Toynbee Hall, which opened in the East End in 1884 following the famous paper that Barnett had read at Oxford the previous November, was based on ideas that had been around for some time (Barnett, 1884). The notion that the privileged ought to go to live among the labouring poor in order to put their time and skills at their disposal, to take up in the towns the position that squires still assumed in rural communities, had been fairly commonplace among the Oxford followers of the moral philosopher T. H. Green. Toynbee Hall (and the other settlements that followed) provided a means by which they could do this, benefit from the support of others engaged in the same work and have access to the resources of an organisation. It is as an agency, one of whose objects was to help the local population acquire organisational skills and resources, that Toynbee Hall can be considered the first community work agency in the country. It was also, significantly enough, a secular version of the traditional church mission among the urban poor, and in that respect a typical product of Green's philosophy which was a sort of secular substitute for Christian theology.

Barnett was so original in many respects that it is nearly half a century before one comes across a community work innovator of anything like comparable stature. Len White's thinking was built not only on his own personal wartime experience in a Pacifist Service Unit but also on the work of the New Estates Committee of the National Council of Social Service (which had done much to promote the idea of community work in new residential areas since its establishment in 1928). He also borrowed extensively from current ideas in town planning. His contribution was to give more systematic form to ideas that were already around and, like Barnett, to show how they could be put into practice.

White worked for some time as a travelling officer on the development of community associations, was a resident community worker on the out-county estate of St Paul's Cray in Kent and later became social development officer at Harlow New Town. Where Barnett's work was based on an apprehension of the problems associated with the rapid growth of London in the nineteenth century, White's thinking was based on an apprehension of the problems associated with urban development in the 1920s and 1930s of this century. Nevertheless, the parallels with Barnett were close in many ways.

White also started from the assumption that classes must exist. The social problems he claimed were evident in the 'tenement towns' and overspill estates were to a large extent the result of a lack of middle-class leadership. The situation represented a moral crisis. We now had 'a rootless generation which has cast off its old traditions and has acquired no new values capable of building a society which will endure' (White, 1950, p. 13). 'The basic problem of the new housing estates' was 'How can such estates become living communities?' (ibid., p. 5). White saw no solution in collective action based on class consciousness. Interclass solidarity built on the basis of interpersonal relationships at the local level provided the key to a social rootedness that recalled all that was best in pre-urban society. White's own action in going to live and work in St Paul's Cray was a personal gesture which he hoped others would imitate. But the longer-term solution depended on the way the environment was planned. White was an enthusiast for the new towns and for design on the basis of 'neighbourhood units' which would incorporate areas of middle-class and working-class housing.

Disillusion with the new towns themselves probably explains why physical planning was undervalued in the thinking of Richard Hauser (1969) who saw a 'crash programme of social education' as the basic solution to problems of urban society, problems he viewed in a similar way to Barnett and White. Hauser's Centre for Group Studies had a tremendous, though not always welcome, impact in certain cities in the period immediately before the recent boom in community work. He was one of a small number of charismatic figures around at the time. But his personal style as well as his conservative, even authoritarian, views made him an increasingly less influential figure in the 1970s.

From the time of Barnett to the late 1960s theories of community work based on a moral vision of neighbourhoods characterised by interclass co-operation dominated community work in this country. When Mayo speaks of the 'catholic and almost mystical sense of community' (1975*a*, p. 8) possessed by Derek Morrell, the civil servant who did much to launch the Home Office Community Development Project, she presumably means to imply that thinking of this sort was significant also in the planning, if not the execution, of the CDP. Since then the dominant tone in British community work has changed. But one can still find those who are in sympathy with older ideals – people such as Phillip Evens who speaks of community work being 'concerned with the pathway to peace in our troubled island' (1974).

Because those who have been considered so far saw community work primarily as a social movement, the notion that it might become a profession is only approached in their writings. It was not until the 1960s that the idea of professional community work was first clearly articulated in the UK, although by the end of the decade it was commonplace, if still controversial.

The origins of this move to professionalism lay in those aspects of the continuing social crisis that were outlined earlier in this chapter. But the immediate ideological origins lay outside Britain itself. In the British colonies of Africa and Asia the twenty years after the Second World War were ones of rapid political change. The major concern of the retreating colonial power was to ensure that, as far as possible, the economic and social patterns that were established in the new nations would be such as to minimise the impact of political independence on the imperialist system. Encouragement was given to development and the creation of political structures that would ensure stability and continuing ties with the motherland. New initiatives in adult education and economic administration were produced under such names as 'basic education', 'extension work' and 'community development' that were paralleled and imitated in other colonial empires and the backward areas of more developed nations.

It has been asserted by the Political Economy Collective of the CDP (1976, p. 1) that colonial 'community development' had an important impact on domestic policy makers, and influenced, for example, the thinking behind the CDP itself. It would probably be more accurate to say that there were analagous attitudes to both the indigenous populations of the colonies and the urban poor in Britain. But there are instances of direct influence. The notable example is that of Dr T. R. Batten who, after lengthy service overseas, became a significant figure in British community work in the 1960s. He first came to prominence with a book on community development overseas (1957). Through his work on training he began to reach a gradually wider audience (1962, 1965), but it was his general textbook published in 1967 that became for a while the most widely used book on courses training social workers, and others for posts in the UK. This outlined a 'non-directive approach' that was similar in many ways to the school of thought on ethical issues that was becoming dominant in the social work profession. It thus offered a bridge for those few theorists who did see lessons in the colonial experience for urban policy in the metropolitan countries. Batten also acted as a consultant to several agencies and retains a significant position as chairman of the editorial board of the *Community Development Journal*, the nearest thing British community work has to a respectable, academic journal.

Among the agencies for which Batten acted as consultant was the North Kensington Family Study Project, with which he became involved on the initiative of its community worker Ilys Booker. She was one of a small number of fieldworkers in the 1960s who gave the incipient notion of community work a clearer character than it could ever have gained from the advocacy of academics such as Phillip Seed, who promoted a number of early discussions on training, or R. A. B. Leaper whose introductory textbook (1971), though widely used for a while, was based scarcely at all on British experience. Ilys Booker was probably the most influential of them all. Born in Canada, she first entered the community work field as an adult educationist in Ontario. She moved to London in the 1950s, joining the staff of the London Council of Social Service. There she was one of those who created a strategy based on a willingness to work with those groups people wanted to form rather than working to the sort of neighbourhood model advocated by White. In 1960–1 she spent eighteen months working for the Danilo Dolci organisation, an experience that confirmed her view that community development should be governed by essentially the same principles in both underdeveloped and developed societies: that it should be a professional activity, non-directive in method and aiming at long-term, slowly accomplished change (Booker, 1962).

Back in England she felt an increasing interest in applying the lessons she felt she had learnt in a few chaotic months in Sicily to a single neighbourhood in London. In 1964 she accepted the post of community worker on the North Kensington Family Study Project and was still in post when she died four years later. Throughout her career in the UK, but especially in the last couple of years, she was an energetic writer of reports and giver of talks. She made initial notes for a basic textbook, but did not get very far with that project. The medium of the talk or lecture was probably more natural to her than that of a full-length book. Her influence derived as much from her personality as from the value people found in what she was saying. She did, however, make a background contribution to two of the first textbooks to be based on practice in Britain (Goetschius, 1969; Mitton and Morrison, 1972).

At a time when many were fascinated by half-comprehended reports on experiences abroad (US community organisation, colonial community development, adult education in the Netherlands, Muintir na Tire in Ireland) Ilys Booker provided a coherent view of community work based on experience in a British city. Her influence in shaping the notion that there was a relevant professional discipline that might be called 'community work' was immense.

But it was a group rather than an individual that brought wider attention to that idea. The term 'community work' itself was coined by a study group founded by the Gulbenkian Foundation (Gulbenkian Foundation, 1968). They saw community work as consisting of three interrelated forms of activity – community development, community organisation and social planning. All three offered solutions to certain modern problems, but they were solutions of a professional nature. While the existence and even value of conflict were acknowledged, they saw the possibility of an overriding consensus. In this they reflected one of the common myths of the 1960s, that all social problems are essentially problems of 'communication'. With their wide-ranging view as to how the term 'community work' should be employed, they acknowledged its relationship to many existing professions and there was a strong education lobby within the group. Nevertheless, the feeling that emerged as dominant was that community work had a special relationship with social work, a view that Ilys Booker had held. This was a reflection of the parallel between some existing casework and community work theory (on non-directiveness, etc.), but also involved recognition of the fact that social work had just 'arrived' as a profession, so that it would be easier to find a niche there than within some more clearly defined profession. At the same time they saw a need for community work to be a specialism and their proposals for training were in line with that conclusion.

The Gulbenkian Report crystallised ideas on community work, and its publication was possibly the most important single event in producing the boom that occurred in the early 1970s. Although there was some resistance to this new-fangled idea, there were many important figures in the social work profession that did their best to promote active interest in it. Leissner's work in relation to family advice centres offered a practical and thought-through example of how community work and casework practice could be related (Leissner, 1967; Leissner *et al.*, 1971). David Jones, principal of the National Institute of Social Work (NISW), played a part in several significant initiatives. He was the first chairman of the Association of Community Workers (ACW), a participant in the various study groups established by the Gulbenkian Foundation, and in the working group on community work training set up by the Central Council for Education and Training in Social Work (CCETSW) (1974), a co-editor of the readers on community work produced by ACW (Jones and Mayo, 1974, 1975) and an important background figure in NISW's Southwark Project which is described by Thomas (1976).

The major obstacle to the acceptance of community work as a part of social work was not a lack of welcoming allies in social work itself, but an increasing resistance to this identification among community workers themselves. There were many reasons for this (including the key role played by adult educationists and youth workers in community work), but it was part of a general anti-professional trend.

Those, such as Batten, Booker, Leissner and the authors of the first Gulbenkian Report who advocated in the 1960s a more professional approach to community work, were responsible for an ideological break with the earlier theorists of community work, such as Barnett, White and Hauser. Although their radical commitment was at best a moderate one, they rejected the explicit conservatism of the earlier activists. Perhaps the best example of this is not the authors already cited, but one of the participants in the Bristol Project that took place in the 1950s and was later described by Spencer (1964). Norman Dennis was among the most caustic debunkers of the 'neighbourhood/community idea' (1958, 1963) and the author of some candid (and instructive) observations on conflict rather than co-operation within community associations (1961).

This breach with open conservatism facilitated the radical trend in British community work in the 1970s. But that radicalism soon went far beyond the moderate reformism of the professionally minded. It has been one of the notable features of British community work in the last few years that it has lacked the sort of advocate of 'radical professionalism' that the USA has had in Gilbert and Specht with their work on participation in the model cities programme (1975) and their 'manifesto' on the 'incomplete profession' of social work (1977). Specht's attempts to put across his views in the UK fell rather flat for several reasons, including the fact that they indicated the extent to which he himself suffered from misconceptions of the British scene (Specht, 1975, 1976).

A rather different and more extreme form of radicalism than that of Specht held the stage in Britain in the early 1970s. It did not necessarily describe the actual practice of the majority of practitioners in the field, but it did to a large extent dominate debate. A key role in the elaboration of this radical approach was played by some of the field staff in the Home Office CDP. Some of the things they had to say were anticipated by Marris and Rein (1967) in their comments on the American poverty programmes. But, being based on American experience, that book had a more restricted influence than some of the publications of the British CDP. The CDP local teams experienced the immediate, small-scale and intimate working conditions of small voluntary agencies, while having a distinct link with government at local and national level. They thus had an impulse to think out the political implications of their work without being subjected to the deadening effect of living within a large bureaucracy. They also had unusual access to publishing facilities.

The first major statement of the position was made by John Benington, project leader in Coventry, at the 1972 ACW conference (Benington, 1972). He raised several basic issues. By concentrating on one area were they, perhaps, helping to stigmatise it? Could the amount of capital they were putting into the area (large by many community workers' standards, but still modest in the light of real needs) make any effective difference? Were they by mediating between local groups and the local authority merely defusing protest or at any rate channelling it into directions acceptable to those in power. Similarly, were they supplying information that would be used by the authority to the advantage or disadvantage of the residents in the target area?

The Benington thesis had a devastating impact and this explains why there is some reaction against it today. After all, it seemed to leave community workers as such with nothing to do. This criticism has been made by one research worker with a CDP team that took a rather different line (Corina, 1977, p. 55). To an extent their own answer was to cease to try to understand the poor and to study the enemy instead. They wrote about the ways in which 'urban deprivation' was a by-product of capitalist growth, of the profits made out of housing, of the limits of the law, of the ways in which local authorities were, in Marx's phrase, 'executive committees of the bourgeoisie' (Community Development Project, 1977*a*, 1977*b*, 1977*c*; Benington, 1976). The theory behind the particular studies was, of course, Marxist, though it was a rather empirical sort of Marxism, providing a series of examples of exploitation rather than developing a Marxist theory of poverty and urban deprivation.

The CDP had a strong research element built into it, so that the production of reports could be justified. A similar line was less open to others who were impressed by the Benington thesis. There were, besides, reasons for supporting community action that were acceptable even to a Marxist placing orthodox emphasis on the primacy of production. Some of these were indicated by Mayo (1975*b*), herself one of the leftists in the CDP. And, if there is a place for community action, there is presumably some place, in at least more favourable situations, for paid community workers. Gradually this conviction has grown. As the first major statement by Benington was made at an ACW conference, it was, perhaps, appropriate that one of the first criticisms of his position to be made from an explicitly socialist perspective should have been offered at the 1977 conference of the association. Smith says with some justification, 'In place of a libertarian naivety about the possibilities of spontaneous change, Marxists have substituted a doctrine of radical pessimism.' He describes their emphasis on 'political education' as 'something of a soft option . . . Such an approach might be more convincing if community workers had really tried; instead I suspect that Marxism has been seized on as a convenient excuse, a dubious explanation for our lack of success.' He finds that 'where the Marxist view taxes my credulity most is in its assumption that community work is putting the lid on working class revolt' and asks for evidence. Finally, he points out that 'most Marxists accept reform as part of the wider struggle . . . For some reason, however, this view of reformist action has not been applied to community work. I suspect, in fact, that at least part of the reason is that community work has in the past made such grandiose claims for itself, so that Marxists have concentrated on redressing the balance' (1978, p. 5).

It is doubtful whether Smith in his paper is as clear on the issue of the relationship between paid community workers and community action as he needs to be. But his assessment of the impact of the CDP Marxists on British community work has much to recommend it. The issue of the relationship between paid staff and community action does, however, remain. This section has dealt mainly with ideas. While these were in debate the creation of community work structures proceeded, though in a somewhat shambling manner.

THE DEVELOPMENT OF COMMUNITY WORK AS A DISTINCT SPHERE OF ACTIVITY

It was a characteristic of social work from its effective beginnings that professional (in the sense of paid) staff were essential to it. At first the paid staff in the COS were mere agents of the middle-class volunteers. But, even at that early stage in the history of social work, the paid agents rapidly assumed a key position in the day-to-day running of the organisation. Of course, caseworkers had an evident function in the smooth running of things. Community work was always a dodgy proposition even when its ideology was impeccably conservative. Thus, although there were paid community workers in settlements, in community centres, in some of the new towns and in various *ad hoc* projects in the period from the founding of Toynbee Hall to the publication of the Gulbenkian Report, their appointment was to deal with particular situations, not part of some generalised move to create a community work service. The situation in social work on which the Seebohm Committee reported (1968) was the natural product of a long period of development. The Gulbenkian Study Group were proposing something that in institutional terms was essentially new.

It is interesting that some twenty years before the Gulbenkian Report was published, there was another report which some expected to have a similar impact, but which failed in the event to do so. In 1949, at a time when there was much interest in the 'neighbourhood/community idea' and the provision of community centres, the Ministry of Education produced what some considered to be a 'charter for neighbourhood workers' (Ministry of Education, 1949; Davies, 1949). The whole movement fitted in with the Labour government's rather muddled egalitarian ideas and, after all, Attlee himself had been at Toynbee Hall. But in the end it all came to nothing. The interest in the neighbourhood-as-community was a mutedly hysterical response to the upheavals of the previous two decades and it became less attractive as the nation drifted into a new period of affluence and self-chosen mobility. It was not the agencies that might be linked to the theoretical perspectives of Barnett and White that provided the basis for the real formation of community work as a distinct entity. It was projects on the fringe of the welfare scene that linked to the perspectives of the more professionally minded theorists – the creation of the Association of London Housing Estates by staff at the London Council of Social Service, the Bristol Project, work with neighbourhood groups in Liverpool in the late 1960s or the more headline-catching activities of such Messianic figures as Hauser on the one hand, and George Clark and other veterans of CND on the other.

The years 1968 and 1969 saw a whole series of reports and initiatives to foster a new interest in community work. The report of the Gulbenkian Study Group was the most important instance. But the Seebohm Report also talked of aspects of community work within the proposed new social services departments (Seebohm, 1968). In the same year the Race Relations Act was passed, providing the legislative basis for the work of community relations councils, and the Urban Programme was launched. In 1969 the Skeffington Report on participation in planning came out, together with a Youth Service Development Council report that said little new, but provided justification for new directions in the youth service, while the Home Office launched the ill-fated Community Development Project (Skeffington, 1969; Youth Service Development Council, 1969).

These initiatives coincided with expressions of interest in community work in several professions. Some of this interest was engendered by academic work that was relevant to but not explicitly about community work and had attracted wide attention in the previous decade. The books produced by the Institute of Community Studies, which suggested an approach to neighbourhood life and organisation rather different from that of White, was one major example. Another was the 'rediscovery' of poverty. A few individuals, such as Peter Townsend, were connected with both these areas of work.

By the mid-1970s there were many new community work posts, and the majority of these were within agencies that had either not existed before or had changed radically. Social services departments were particularly important. But community education sections in education departments were also making a new contribution within local authorities. In the non-statutory sector the most significant single new agency was the Young Volunteer Force Foundation, which, in the light of its changing function, has recently restyled itself the Community Projects Foundation. There were also many local projects, some within councils of social service, others set up on a more *ad hoc* basis, many of them funded to a significant extent from new forms of central government grant aid. Community work as it is practised in those agencies, community work as we know it today, has its origins in a loose sense in the history that stretches back to Barnett, but more specifically in the sudden spurt of interest in 1968–9.

The factors that made 1968 a watershed are not difficult to locate. There was, first of all, the growing dissatisfaction with the evident limitations to the peaceful 'revolution' of 1968. 'Participation' initiated and managed by community workers seemed one answer among many to the problems of 'distant and anonymous authority' (Gulbenkian, 1968, p. 4).

Then there was another effect of the continuing growth of the welfare state. It had meant the gradual expansion of new professions that resented the bureaucratic limitations of the organisations that had enabled them to expand, particularly in local government. Community work offered to discontented radicals in welfare services a new specialism, a radical alternative and various other tempting goodies. This was particularly true of social work, and it is not surprising that social services departments have provided the single most important growth point for employment opportunities.

A third reason was that, again with the continuing growth of the welfare state, there were rising expectations that met headlong the increasing inability of government to cope. The initiatives of 1968–9 took place against a background that included rent strikes in almost every major city as council rents went up and rebate schemes became more and more common in the run-up to the 1972 Housing Finance Act. Coincidentally, the slum-clearance programmes of many cities, having run through the worst older housing, came up against areas where older housing was often owner-occupied and suitable for improvement. To the amazement, even downright incredulity, of many Labour councillors, people began to protest against proposed demolition. The issues relating to housing found parallels elsewhere. There was a new attitude abroad to claiming the 'charity' of the state that led to the formation of claimants' unions and other groups concerned partly or entirely with state benefits that were organised, not by concerned professionals (as the Child Poverty Action Group had largely been), but by claimants themselves. This new rebellion was important to community work in two ways. It created a problem that the authorities needed to manage (so that new posts were established), and it attracted into community work people who wanted to encourage such forms of activity.

A fourth reason was that community work was able to provide an apparent – even at times prestigious – solution to social problems at comparatively little cost. The CDP leftists claimed that the various poverty experiments which dated mainly from the 1968–9 period were an exercise in 'gilding the ghetto' (CDP, 1977*d*). Similar criticism might be levelled against some local authorities who went in for community work on a comparatively large scale. To provide adequate resources for domiciliary services in a neighbourhood might cost a fortune and gain little attention beyond a grumble from the local ratepayers' association. A tin-pot project employing a couple of young, low-paid enthusiasts working from a disused shop might have the capacity to gain favourable coverage in the professional press as an 'imaginative' venture and even be sufficiently photogenic to make it on telly. With increasing cutbacks in local authority spending, community work was among the first to suffer in many places, being regarded by councillors as either a luxury or a pain in the neck. Yet even in recent years community projects have often been established as a cheap alternative to more comprehensive services – the financial assistance of the Manpower Services Commission often being the source of temptation.

Although the 1971–2 boom in community work employment has flattened out, the consequences of it have not yet clearly emerged. Community work is still at the end of its beginning. But something of the consequent unclarity about the nature of community work can be seen in the very restricted extent to which community work's own institutions have developed to keep pace with the increase in posts.

The resplendently titled Association of Community Workers in the United Kingdom was formed as a result of discussions in 1968 by people who wished to establish a new professional association that might, perhaps, become assimilated by the proposed British Association of Social Workers. Criticism from the new radicals in community work within and outside ACW led it to drop its pretensions to represent a new profession in 1973 when it opened up its membership to anyone prepared to accept its general objectives. This change did nothing to protect it from an increasing loss of membership over the following three years, a trend it shared with the professional associations with which it had parted company. ACW never developed a branch structure, in spite of the fact that local community workers' groups flourished at least in the larger cities, and this failure condemned it to relative ineffectiveness. In 1976 it decided to reorganise itself as a kind of federation of local networks of community workers. In spite of initial enthusiasm, development in this direction has been slow or non-existent in all but a few places.

Parallel development took place in the field of training. The Gulbenkian Report had been primarily about training and had made recommendations on the subject, but these failed to produce a coherent policy because there was no centre to direct such a policy. Meanwhile among fieldworkers there was a growing demand for training to be at the initiative of regional training groups (covering areas larger than the networks of fieldworkers) which would be autonomous and concerned with their own zone of influence. Co-ordination and development was entrusted to a body significantly named as the 'Interim Central Group' as the result of a conference at Manchester in January 1977.

Although no institution was empowered to take the initiative in the development of structures at national level to service community work, initiative of a sort did remain with the group that had produced the Gulbenkian Report. The Gulbenkian Foundation (which also played an important role by funding local projects, particularly in the fields of community art and education) offered financial support to a new group under the chairmanship of Lord Boyle which included many of the original group. This new group produced a useful overview of the community work scene (Gulbenkian Community Work Group, 1973) which among other things suggested the need for a national resource centre and a national forum on community work. The national resource centre proposal became the victim of the financial recession. The Gulbenkian Foundation set up a second successor to the original group (again with some of the original members) as an advisory committee on its work with resource centres at local level. This committee attempted to revive the notion of a national forum at a conference held in Birmingham in January 1977, but the hostility expressed by some fieldworkers (particularly through ACW) was so great that the advisory committee retreated.

The debate on the 'forum' proposal may be seen as marking the rejection by community workers themselves of their identity as the product of a liberal movement of opinion within the establishment. But, if the alleged 'élitism' and 'centralism' of the forum proposal was rejected, what was to take its place? Were the community workers in ACW arguing for their right to organise their own profession in the way that social workers had done, or were they arguing for something different? And, if so, what? Or were they arguing against centralism on the basis of some kind of anarchistic principle that power should rest with autonomous groups small enough to operate on a face-to-face basis? For all their accusations that the advisory committee was vague in its proposals, it is not obvious what were ACW's answers to these questions. The protest against the 'forum', like the moves in favour of 'devolved' forms of organisation for training and for ACW itself were, above all, indicators of the ambiguity of community work's status, or lack of status, as a profession.

COMMUNITY WORK ON THE BOUNDARIES OF PROFESSIONALISM

It is practically received opinion that professionalism is a bulwark of conservatism. Unfortunately for that viewpoint, there is a good deal of evidence that 'professionalism' measured in certain ways is likely to have the opposite effect, Epstein's research on New York social workers being the best example (Epstein, 1969, 1970).

There is evidently some confusion here and the confusion arises from the way that sociologists have chosen to define professionalism. They have sought to render the concept more specific by translating it into operational terms. This is useful for some purposes, but has the effect of de-historicising the terms of the discussion. Actual professions are investigated to see what are their major characteristics. Whether an occupation is more or less a profession and whether a practitioner is more or less professional in his outlook or behaviour can then be measured according to the number and strength of the characteristics shown. 'Professionalism' becomes a quality which can exist in greater or lesser measures. But this is not what it is in fact. It is part of an historical process. Bearing this in mind, one can distinguish three types of profession. These all have characteristics in common, because they are all part of the process of the evolution of a middle class whose prestige and higher incomes help to blur the line between capital and labour. But it remains important to distinguish them.

The first type is that which tends to be considered professionalism *par excellence*, that of the legal and medical profession. These have a distinct body of knowledge, a virtual monopoly of its use, considerable autonomy and self-government and (in spite of criticism) widely acknowledged high status. The institutional arrangements by which the first set of professions protect their own monopoly have been imitated by the second group whose occupational activity is also based on esoteric knowledge. This group includes professions such as engineering and others with a base in the natural sciences. Although these occupational groups have often succeeded in winning monopolistic positions and high financial rewards for their members, they have failed on the whole to secure high status.

The third set of professions form a quite different group, although it is possible to see some parallels with the first.

The oldest profession is not prostitution but priesthood, and priesthood as we know it in our society (that is the priesthood of the Christian churches) is the key institution in the bureaucratic stabilisation of a social movement. Similarly in England the legal profession first emerged as a significant force in the early seventeenth century when its reinterpretation of existing law (particularly Magna Carta) provided the main ideological weapon of the new middle class against the remnants of the feudal aristocracy. One aspect of professionalism is, therefore, that it can represent an attempt to translate the objectives of a social movement into a set of institutions that can be accommodated within existing society and thereby operate in a routine manner over a period of time. The third set of professions is that in which this characteristic is dominant.

Towards the end of the last century three broad movements of social reform emerged which sought to create institutional structures that would allow for the achievement of their objectives. These were the movements for universal education, for better planning of towns, and for more humane treatment of the poor. By the middle of the present century their efforts (and much stronger forces, themselves responsible for the emergence of these movements in the first place) led to the creation of the welfare state. The movements became the new professions that ran that state – teaching, planning and social work (together with many related professions, such as nursery education and housing management). These professions are social movements transformed by the process of incorporation into the state bureaucracy. Their professionalism is a compromise between movement and bureaucracy.

When comparisons are made between community work and professions of the third group (especially social work) the parallels are obvious. Community work is simply the last arrival on the scene. It is ironic that a social movement that had as one of its origins a distrust of officials should have culminated in the creation of a new type of local government officer – the community worker. But, given the history of social work and planning, this might have been expected. That community work has deviated from the pattern of the third group has been due primarily to the fact that it was the most recent arrival. Having a much less obvious function in the smooth running of things than people who run clear-cut services (such as environmental health inspectors), or people who help organise (such as planners), or even people who tidy away problems (such as social workers), community workers were only invented as a clearly distinct and relatively large-scale group when certain aspects of social organisation appeared to be getting out of hand. But, precisely because of the crisis that was developing, the staff recruited into community work were inclined to reject liberal notions of professionalism that had satisfied most social workers. The reasons why community work experienced a sudden boom in the early 1970s explain the paradox that lies at its centre – that it became hostile to the state at precisely the moment that the state was most prepared to adopt it.

This paradox has led to some confused thinking about community work and professionalism. If a welfare profession is a social movement that has been incorporated into the state (or its associated structures in the voluntary sector), then in that sense community work must be a profession or not exist at all. (Perhaps the dichotomy should not be drawn so sharply. There is a third hypothetical option and that is that community work should receive massive sponsorship from the trade union movement. But there are no signs that this is likely to happen. And, if it did happen, it might well be on the basis of an even closer relationship between union and government than has developed under recent Labour administrations. In that case, the relationship between unions and the state would be much more like that between the larger voluntary organisations and the state, so that the radical potential in trade union sponsorship would be reduced.) There is no question of community workers having the option to be 'professional' (in the sense in which the word is being used here) or not. What they do have the option of doing is accepting or rejecting a professionalist ideology, one that would welcome their incorporation into the state machine because of a reformist belief (such as that of Harry Specht) in the potential of the existing state for the achievement of a maximum feasible degree of well-being.

But between the bare fact of being in practical terms a profession and the acceptance of professionalism as an ideology there is a whole area of ambiguity and uncertainty. Is it possible to secure opportunities for skill development without establishing a professionalist outlook on the question of qualification? Can people in the community work occupation secure adequate salaries without resort to arguments related to professional status?

While community workers rejected any notion that they belonged to a profession, intelligent discussion of this sort of issue was impossible. There was a tendency to drift into an effective ideological professionalism while maintaining an anti-professional rhetoric. Even if this is understood, the answers to the questions do not become easy, and must all be based on intelligent guesses on the likely outcome of particular developments. One element in the construction of a general answer is that community workers should become active trade unionists. This would protect their interests without resort to arguments from professionalism, render them more aware of their own situation and create new opportunities for realising the much discussed need to forge alliances between community groups and trade unions. Other elements might also be suggested. But the questions will always need new answers.

The key boundary in community work is that on which all radical community workers stand between the world of welfare professions in which they gain the means to live and the movement for change to which they belong. To be in the welfare state but not of it is the crucial requirement made of them by the commitment to which they lay claim.

REFERENCES

Barnett, S. A. (1884). *Settlements of University Men in Great Towns*, reprinted in Pimlott, J. A. R. (1935), *Toynbee Hall: Fifty Years of Social Progress 1884–1934* (London: Dent), pp. 266–73.

Batten, T. R. (1957). *Communities and Their Development: An Introductory Study with Special Reference to the Tropics* (London: OUP).

Batten, T. R. (1962). *Training for Community Development: A Critical Study of Method* (London: OUP).

Batten, T. R. with Batten, M. (1965). *The Human Factor in Community Work* (London: OUP).

Batten, T. R. (1967). *The Non-Directive Approach in Group and Community Work* (London: OUP).

Benington, J. (1972). 'Community work as an instrument of institutional change', in *Lessons from Experience* (London: ACW).

Benington, J. (1976). *Local Government Becomes Big Business* (London: CDP Information and Intelligence Unit).

Booker, I. (1962). 'Project in Menfi: an experiment in social development', *Social Services Quarterly*, vol. 35, no. 4.

Community Development Project (1977*a*). *The Costs of Industrial Change* (London: CDP Inter-Project Editorial Team).

Community Development Project (1977*b*). *Profits against Housing* (London: CDP Inter-Project Editorial Team).

Community Development Project (1977*c*). *Limits of the Law* (London: CDP Inter-Project Editorial Team).

Community Development Project (1977*d*). *Gilding the Ghetto: The State and the Poverty Experiments* (London: CDP Inter-Project Editorial Team).

Corinna, L. (1977). *Oldham CDP: An Interim Assessment of Its Impact and Influence on the Local Authority*, Papers in Community Studies No. 9 (University of York).

Davies, A. S. (1949). 'A charter for neighbourhood workers?', *Social Services Quarterly*, vol. 23, no. 2.

Dennis, N. (1958). 'The popularity of the neighbourhood/community idea', *Sociological Review*, new series, vol. 6, no. 1.

Dennis, N. (1961). 'Changes in function and leadership renewal: a study of the community association movement and problems of voluntary small groups in the urban locality', *Sociological Review*, new series, vol. 9, no. 1, pp. 55–84.

Dennis, N. (1963). 'Who needs neighbours?', *New Society* 43. (July).

Engels, F. (1956). *The Housing Question*, 'Marx and Engels Selected Works', Vol. 1 (Moscow: Foreign Languages Publishing House).

Epstein, I. (1969). 'Professionalisation, professionalism and social worker radicalism', *Journal of Health and Social Behaviour* (9 March).

Epstein, I. (1970). 'Specialisation, professionalisation and social worker radicalism: a test of the "process" model of a profession', *Applied Social Studies*, vol. 2.

Evens, P. (ed.) (1974). *Community Work Theory and Practice* (Oxford: Shornach).

Gilbert, N. and Specht, H. (1975). 'Socio-political correlates of community action: conflict, political integration and citizen influence', in P. Leonard (ed.), *The Sociology of Community Action*, Sociological Review Monograph No. 21.

Gilbert, N. and Specht, H. (1977). 'The incomplete profession', in H. Specht and A. Vickery (eds) *Integrating Social Work Methods* (London: Allen & Unwin).

Goetschius, G. (1969). *Working With Community Groups Using Community Development as a Method of Social Work* (London: Routledge).

Gulbenkian Community Work Group (1973). *Current Issues in Community Work* (London: RKP).

Gulbenkian Foundation (1968). *Community Work and Social Change* (London: Longmans).

Hauser, R. (1969). 'The invisible community', in S. Verney (ed.), *People and Cities* (London: Fontana).

Hebditch, S. (1976). 'Ideology of grass roots action', in P. Hain (ed.), *Community Politics* (London: Calder).

Holyoake, G. J. (1893). *Self-Help by the People: The History of the Rochdale Pioneers 1844–1892* (London: Swan Sonnenschein).

Jones, D. and Mayo, M. (eds) (1974). *Community Work: One* (London: Routledge).

Jones, D. and Mayo, M. (eds) (1975). *Community Work: Two* (London: Routledge).

Leaper, R. A. B. (1971). *Community Work: An Introduction* (London: National Council of Social Service).

Leat, D. (1975). 'Social theory and the historical construction of social work activity: the role of Samuel Barnett', in P. Leonard (ed.) *The Sociology of Community Action*, Sociological Review Monograph No. 21.

Leissner, A. (1967). *Family Advice Centres* (London: Longmans).

Leissner, A. *et al.* (1971). *Advice, Guidance and Assistance: A Study of Seven Family Advice Centres* (London: Longmans).

Loch, C. S. (1885). *Seventeenth Annual Report of the Charity Organisation Society* (London: COS).

Marris, P. and Rein, M. (1967). *Dilemmas of Social Reform* (London: Routledge).

Mayo, M. (1975*a*). 'The history and early development of CDP', in R. Lees and G. Smith (eds) *Action Research in Community Development* (London: Routledge).

Mayo, M. (1975*b*). 'Community development: a radical alternative?', in R. Bailey and M. Brake (eds) *Radical Social Work* (London: Arnold).

Mayo, M. (ed.) (1977). *Women in the Community* (London: Routledge).

Ministry of Education (1949). *Report of the Committee on Recruitment, Training and Conditions of Service of Youth Leaders and Community Centre Wardens* (London: HMSO).

Mitton, R. and Morrison, E. (1972). *A Community Project in Notting Dale* (London: Allen Lane).

Nevitt, A. A. (1966). *Housing, Taxation and Subsidies* (London: Nelson).

Political Economy Collective (1976). *Community Work or Class Politics?* (London: CDP).

Seebohm Report (1968). *Report of the Committee on Local Authority and Allied Personal Social Services* (London: HMSO).

Skeffington Report (1969). *People and Planning: Report of the Committee on Public Participation in Planning* (London: HMSO).

Smith, J. (1978). 'Possibilities for a socialist community work practice', in *Towards a Definition of Community Work* (London: ACW).

Specht, H. (1975). *Community Development in the UK: An Assessment and Recommendation for Change* (London: ACW).

Specht, H. (1976). *The Community Development Project: National and Local Strategies for Improving the Delivery of Services* (London: NISW).

Spencer, J. (1964). *Stress and Release in an Urban Housing Estate* (London: Tavistock).

Thomas, D. N. (1976). *Organising for Social Change: A Study in the Theory and Practice of Community Work* (London: Allen & Unwin).
Thomas, J. H. (1920). *When Labour Rules* (London: Collins).
White, L. E. (1950). *Community or Chaos: Housing Estates and Their Social Problems* (London: National Council of Social Service).
Young, G. M. (1953). *Victorian England: Portrait of an Age* (London: OUP).
Youth Service Development Council (1969). *Youth and Community Work in the Seventies* (London: HMSO).

Chapter 2

PRACTICE AND THEORY IN COMMUNITY WORK: A CASE FOR RECONCILIATION

Laurence J. Tasker

The distinction between philosophy and theory is not complete as there seems to be a link-up at some stage in the life of the latter with the former. However, it is necessary to show where one's working definition of a philosophy ends and of a theory begins. Briefly, a philosophical proposition can be taken as an evaluative proposition about any act or thing which cannot be modified by empirical testing. Thus a community worker believes in extending participation because it is an end in itself – an experience intrinsically valuable and central to the concept of 'the good life' which informs the goals of his work. A theoretical proposition is, for example, that increasing public control over local resources is more efficient – i.e. cheaper – than having them professionally managed, or alternatively more likely in the long term to maintain public order.

Theorising is important because it moves practice out of the realm of random speculation and into that of properly reckoned strategy and planning. To some, theorising may seem pretentious and unnecessary because the need for community work is so widespread and so obvious. This chapter is written on the assumptions that the need will not be universally recognised, that community work will have increasingly to compete for resources, and that a better-argued case will help it to do so.

Theorising in community work takes a number of forms:

(1) The first, a familiar kind of theory, is the theory of social policy. This describes where community work fits in an overall strategy of services to and control of society. A community worker has to know how he or she relates to other professions in addition to developing a practice theory. Thus community workers can develop, for example, a knowledge of the political intentions of their employers to be related to the objectives of their own profession. This is the realm of 'policy theory'.

(2) Another kind of theory is provided by the discipline of sociology. It describes the social world in which the community worker acts and the way its different parts relate. In particular it describes culture. Sociology has been developed in Britain with social policy in mind, but it has been concerned with manipulation and direction rather than activation – in particular with the theory of class.

Community workers need a theory indicating the opportunities for intervention and potential for change. They need sociology but with additions to form a dynamic theory – an analysis of change at the micro level. This may be called 'contextual theory'.

(3) Model building represents a kind of theorising which has been common in the social sciences. It produces a provisional pattern which can be used to order observations on social phenomena. Data is thus more easily organised. It does help in providing the boundaries to certain types of phenomena. This is true of community work and has aided the definitions of professional and related tasks. It does not attempt to produce 'if . . . then' propositions concerning day-to-day practice, but helps the community worker understand his task more clearly in terms of policy theory. Such theories will be called 'models'.

(4) If community workers understand the boundaries of their professional role, where it fits in social policy, and the community in which they are going to work, they still need to know what happens if they adopt a certain kind of practice. This is the most important kind of theorising in community work. A great deal of technique has become available from the wide and varied experience of recent years, and it has to be assessed and the various questions of effectiveness and consequence answered. This is the task of building up a 'practice theory' in community work.

Ideas current in community work practice will be discussed within these four categories. Reliance will not be placed solely on the literature of community work as this does not always reflect adequately the state of thought in the profession and current ideas must be judged sometimes in an *ad hoc* fashion.

This typology is, of course, a 'model' in itself and the theories discussed will not necessarily fall neatly into any one category. In fact, the bias of the argument will fall towards practice theories, and ideas which might have been included in other categories are considered in that section for their practice implications. The tenor of the chapter is avowedly speculative. The aim is as much to stimulate theorising as to review it.

POLICY THEORIES

John Benington (1974) wrote 'Strategies for change at the local level' on the basis of less than three years' experience at Coventry Community Development Project (CDP). Soon after, the central team of CDP published a similar argument in 'Forward Plan' (National Community Development Project, 1975). It was argued that local analysis of social deprivation was not enough. Community work, if it was to be useful, had to be part of a strategy. Poverty, though manifested at a local level, was a national phenomenon and the solutions needed to be calculated likewise. Thus a community worker had to have a concept of his or her work not only *vis-à-vis* a local population, but as part of a national policy or movement. In a single chapter it is impossible to assess the possibilities of policy theorising itself, but it remains important to echo Benington and the lessons of CDP regarding the attitudes of community workers to macro analysis. Community workers' main work is face to face with the recipients, which makes macro-level perspectives difficult; yet to fail to adopt one is to risk disappointment, as was experienced by so many after the CDP programme. There is a great temptation in a helping profession to preoccupy oneself with the individual person. Policy makers, however, do not suffer this constraint, and they direct welfare services according to well-thought-out policy theories of their own. To fail to do likewise on the part of community workers incurs two risks. First, they fail to match their own arguments for the provision of the service against those put forward elsewhere in public and professional life. Secondly, they risk manipulation through a lack of awareness of the type of scheme into which their projects are intended to fit. In fact community workers need to be better social-policy theorists than others because of the extreme political sensitivity surrounding their profession.

Policy theories and ideologies can be very close to each other. Community workers tend to be good at the second and less articulate in the first. The reason may be found partly in training. A paper on training which promises to be very influential has recently been circulated by the Central Council for Education and Training in Social Work (1978).

In the discussion of 'relevant degrees' for social work training there is no mention of the special requirements of community work. Moreover, there is no discussion of political science in any context as a relevant social science subject. To this must be added the general observation that for many social work training courses the study of welfare institutions comes under the heading 'social administration' rather than 'social policy'. These may appear synonymous but, essentially, they are not. An analytical approach to welfare administration is a theoretical and empirical discussion of policy implementation, whereas the social administration of so many courses concerns the mechanical functions of different agencies and a historical perspective on the welfare state. This does not stimulate the kind of theorising which social workers and community workers trained in those circumstances require. The result is a narrow, micro-oriented approach to their profession.

An institution which can help a profession to articulate its ideas on social policy, consolidate these among its members, and encourage this kind of awareness is a professional association. Unfortunately attitudes to this idea have not been at all encouraging in community work. This seems rather short-sighted. As Teresa Smith suggests in Chapter 13, professional organisation has been resisted because it suggests élitism, protectionism, de-skilling the client, and so on. It has thus not adequately been considered for its potential to protect principles, and provide a countervailing power to those who would manipulate community work to other ends. The Association of Community Workers has represented the main attempt to overcome this, but remains thwarted by the ambivalence of potential members and their dispersal in a variety of other professional associations and unions. Community work has thus lost another aid to the development and consolidation of its theories about social policy and a voice to advocate its own place within them.

There is also a kind of voluntarism current in community work which actually resists identification with a wider movement or separate analysis. It sees the 'helping' of the helping professions as adequate justification for its existence, and political or quasi-political analysis as corrupting of the spirit. Hopefully, this narrowness is dying out faster in community work than in other professions; this may be due to some excellent critical texts directed at the 'liberal' position (Mayo, 1975; Cockburn, 1977). Theories replacing those which this approach challenges are, however, hard to find in the literature. For example there is much to be done in clearly locating community work in a Marxist, or any other, theory of social change. Further, the partly spelt-out and rather confused theory of community work exampled in the Seebohm Report has never been completely consolidated.

One is faced, therefore, with an inadequate level of policy theorising in community work. Neither the training system nor professional organisation within community work are geared to establishing a tradition of thought at that level, and the wave of negative comment following the disappointment with the CDP still needs complementing with sound theory construction. Unlike other levels of theorising, where the appeal is to individual initiative, the level of analysis here

– like that of the theories it concerns – are macro in dimension. Only through changes in the traditions of the profession will real improvement be achieved.

MODELS

The tradition of model building in community work has its origins firmly in the social sciences as developed in the USA. Models are a means of organising ideas and formulating categories in a new discipline. Community work has likewise featured a great deal of model building in its literature, possibly due to American influence. In fact, models probably present the greatest theoretical preoccupation in community work so far. The reasons for this are difficult to reckon, but certainly involve the boundary issues in establishing a new profession and the related problem of impressing policy-makers with a clear identity. This preoccupation with definition has tended to mask some of the theoretical issues raised in model building.

The construction of models in community work may be broadly categorised in two types: the more articulate, carefully delineated models concerned with range and definitions in practice; and the second, which may be implied as well as explicit, concerned with the professional definition of the task or of the worker, The first, including Gulbenkian Foundation (1968), Rothman (1974), Thomas (1975), Leissner (1975) and Norris (1977), tend to be indirectly concerned with practice theory. For example, Leissner appears concerned to present a clear pattern of categories of community work practice to employing authorities, and Norris offers a typology whereby community workers may categorise their own practice. The limitation of these analyses is perhaps illustrated by Thomas who goes beyond this aim by arguing some of the practice implications in his model, i.e. in the type of leadership different varieties of action produce. Models of the second sort concerning, for example, the community worker as group worker (Klein, 1963) or social planner (Thomas, 1978) tend, like the former type, to feature mainly an indirect concern with practice theory.

Outstanding matters in model building include such 'boundary issues' as the question of community organisation's place in delineating community work practice. This is part of the traditional model of community work practice in Britain, but it is open to question as to whether interagency co-ordination work, for example on behalf of a local authority, can be counted in the same job definition as the grass-roots work involving very basic initiating carried out by many fieldworkers. For many, community work has come virtually to mean neighbourhood work. Undoubtedly community organisation – in the British sense of the expression – is an important skill in neighbourhood work, but it hardly characterises it. On the other hand, interagency work almost exclusively makes up the task of some workers who are still inclined to be regarded as community workers. The bases of the jobs are so different as to make it doubtful that the same job label is appropriate. It may also be undesirable for community work to have its definitions left thus wide unless there is clarity of the identity of such fundamentals as, for example, technical skills or educational aims. Such obscurity does not help clarify aims and without clarity of aims practice theory cannot mature.

Confrontationist concepts involved in such elements of job models as 'community action' and 'social action' tend more clearly to imply concepts of practice theory. Confrontationist tactics may be deduced from a conflict analysis of society and be seen as the best practice method to make that clear. They may also be adopted for their relation to other aims in practice. A few writers, notably Bryant (1972), have treated community action with a view to practice theory, but in general in has received little such analysis. The consequences of such a tactic in terms of, say, effect on neighbourhoods, the stability of organisations, the standing of the worker, patterns of leadership, and the relating of these to alternative tactics, that is alternative parts of the same model, warrant a great deal of further discussion. More data and improved empirical testing may become indispensible for such an analysis to progress.

Related to the question of social action in such models is the influence of American writing in this branch of theorising, introducing a point of contextual theory. A model is more intent on establishing categories than the relationships between them. Thus a dimension such as social action may appear in a British model of community work but have far less practical significance than its American counterpart. Alinsky (1969) inspired many British community workers of the 1960s with his highly confrontationist and apparently successful approach. That such scenarios did not occur in quite the same way here is due to the essential differences between American and British politics. American politics are more pluralist in nature, especially at city level, meaning an openness to new initiatives and response to the representation of interest groups. In Britain they are more institutionalised and less flexible. Thus a model may be complete by the inclusion of such categories, but have limited usefulness in indicating applicability or consequences in practice.

Models of the second type mentioned above are perhaps more polemical due to their concerns with job definitions and professional boundaries, but have done much to stimulate discussion about the types of skills involved in community work. Because of their concern with skills, however, they have implications for practice, and could be considered more in these terms than simply interprofessional debate, thus advancing the development of practice theory.

It would be pretentious and unjust to draw generalisations about models without a very thorough review. They have doubtless had a usefulness beyond adequate analysis here. However, they are not so divorced from the cause and effect notions of practice theory as might appear. They have generally been constructed looking 'upwards' rather than 'downwards' and this has undoubtedly been their chief contribution. However, there is scant reminder in these structures of the effects on individual people which is ultimately what community work is about. A shift to the analysis of theoretical propositions within models might now be a timely development.

CONTEXTUAL THEORY

Understanding of the social context of such an undertaking as community work might rightfully be expected to fall within the province of sociology. Unfortunately the British tradition of sociology, in as far as it has been directed towards social policy, has appeared to treat underprivileged communities with a view to highlighting their various features for better administration rather than for their potential to change. The tradition of class analysis tends to treat the phenomena of working-class areas with an almost patronising detachment, praising features only when they appear to generate some internal support system, which otherwise – it might not too cynically be argued – might be a burden on the rates. Even Hoggart (1957) – giving an example of an 'inside' approach – leaves an impression of near apology, or at best nostalgia, but not advocacy. None of these academics seemed concerned to evaluate features of working-class life for their intrinsic merit, and still less for their potential to self-generated change. This is the limit on the usefulness of sociological analysis to the community worker, where he or she as a practitioner has to add to its theory. Sociology is conventionally a static analysis; community work is a dynamic practice, that is, it is oriented to change. While the data of sociology is indispensable, the theory of context in community work needs to be a dynamic one, and therefore to build up additional knowledge of its own.

There are many features of working-class life where this kind of theorising is necessary. The following example stands out from among recently prominent aspects of the theory of practice in the profession:

A theory of communications in community work has to take into account certain differences which are apparent across class boundaries. Industry, requiring a large workforce, also requires housing for that workforce which thus tends to be located nearby. The result is that associations in the geographical community are often transcended and supported by parallel associations in the workplace. This greatly improves the informal organisational potential among such people. Moreover, geographical proximity itself produces advantages from a communications point of view. Women, when housebound, tend to experience a high degree of direct contact, and relative absence of personal transport and localisation of facilities tends to increase this. More important, the tendency for families to stay together geographically provides a natural system of communication links, though the actual significance of this in practice remains unclear.

On the negative side it may be noted that working-class districts have fewer telephones and cars. These material disadvantages may to some extent be counter-balanced by the advantages mentioned above. In any event, it seems that the community worker should capitalise on the advantages presented.

This leads to a question relating to one device in community work, namely the formal meeting. Earlier texts appeared to assume that formal meetings were the primary organisational device in community work and large tracts of analyses were given over to conducting them. Although these obviously have a place at a certain stage of community work this is unlikely, ideally, to be an early stage. It should be remembered that in addition to the obvious ones mentioned above there is the more subtle cultural factor that formal meetings may be very intimidating. This will particularly be the case where the location is in a sense hostile, such as a school or even church hall. House meetings gain very little attention in the literature and one wonders how far this is reflected by their actual usage in practice. In any event, it seems they may have the potential to replace a great deal of the formal organisational side of community work through avoiding the inhibition of environment and procedure. Formal organisation is an inevitable end of community work but an unnecessarily prominent means.

The place of formal organisation in community work practice is chosen because it involves a number of examples of contextual theory. Very relevant in this respect is the notion of apathy and aspects of political culture which are associated with it. This is discussed elsewhere (Tasker, 1978). A more obvious point where sociology can be informative is in the relationship between leisure activity and formal organisations. Briefly, 'joining' is a more middle-class phenomenon, and working-class recreational preferences do not feature formal organised activity so strongly (Reid, 1977, pp. 219–21). This has implications for the community worker, obviously, in the type and style of recreational activities he or she encourages. More generally, it limits the extent to which the community worker can expect enthusiasm for formal organisational activity, even of an instrumental or political nature. Working-class people may not actually like meetings, whereas, to risk a caricature, middle-class people may be said often to make a pastime of them.

A further feature of this cultural difference is its relationship to the time dimension of the theory of organisations. There is a tendency in community work to aim for the stable durable organisation, for example the tenants' association, which can safeguard the interests of an area on a long-term basis. Clearly this has many advantages and a complete analysis is not intended here. But durable multi-purpose organisations may not be the most conducive to community work's aims in working-class communities. If attitudes to organised, self-protective activity and skill in carrying this out is a basic aim, this might better be effected through ephemeral, issue-centred activity. This may 'go against the grain' instinctively and it is easy to overstate the case, but one frequently hears disillusionment when an organisation 'folds' and the reasoning behind this disappointment is seldom clearly stated. The short-term success may have more benefit in educational terms than long-term, organisation-centred effort. The educational versus material aims of community work may be at issue here; for example, there is little choice but to mount a long-term, organised campaign with a stable core of individuals to direct it in the case of a planning dispute. Often, though, the preference for conventional organisation may be more in the sentiments of the workers than in the rationale of their practice.

The central concept of organisation is therefore shown to be a lot more problematic when it is related to the culture where a project is to take place. Other cultural features need to be treated with similar seriousness. For example, vandalism was not found to be such an important 'problem' to one neighbourhood as it was in the local city hall. When all else had failed cash was given to community groups in the area to find a solution. It was found a year later that they had not spent the money on this at all, but on play schemes for young children and old people's welfare. These were much more important, it was said. Only when customs and values of a community and their relation to practice theories are understood can the potential for change within it really be evaluated.

PRACTICE THEORY

Commitment to a practice theory of community work means facing up to difficulties of a scientific nature. The distinguishing feature of a theory is that it is testable, but in relation to community work testing poses methodological problems. For example, a project's effect on an area might be very difficult to measure in terms of quality of life or marginal political awareness. Sociology may catch up with this kind of problem in the techniques it has to offer; meanwhile community workers may have to develop better *ad hoc* judgements of effectiveness – or at least more systematic ones – to enhance their own methods and consolidate their status among other social services.

The following are examples of issues current in practice theory.

The Role of Organisations

Crucial to community work practice theory is the role of organisations. Often these are overtly political organisations such as action groups. Just as frequent, however, are the non-political organisations encouraged by community workers such as play associations, old people's recreational clubs, and so on. Many community workers work on the assumption that organising has a politicising effect, and such organisations as the latter have a place in community work not just for the service they provide but because they develop a predisposition to participate politically in the more general sense. That politically relevant skills – such as organising and committee work – are imparted is pretty well indisputable. However, the proposition that such activity results in increased political behaviour is testable and has been the subject of some research in sociology and political science.

Ziblatt (1963) studied the predispositions of some American adolescents to participate politically in relation to their organised leisure-time activities. His research did not show this predisposition to be affected, though this may have been a function of his research instrument as other findings seemed to bear out the community work theory: organised leisure activity gave a 'feeling of integration' which led to a 'positive' attitude to politics. Another American researcher had earlier produced similar results (Newcomb, 1943). Although the correlations in these pieces of research may not be so distinct as hoped, community work method seems basically to be borne out. Survey method, however, is not now relied upon so exclusively in sociology, and the more favoured case study might produce better results in this respect, and at the same time be more amenable to community workers' collecting their own information.

The Neighbourhood Effects

Another point of theory, by contrast, presents methodological problems of a more intractable nature. This is the idea that a piece of community activity, if sufficiently spectacular, will take effect on the neighbourhood in which it occurs. A community festival may be seen to affect general morale in a district (Hoyland, 1976). More usually, a piece of political confrontation such as a squat – if well publicised –

is seen to raise political consciousness among the surrounding population. A demonstration is a more obvious example. The effect under discussion is sometimes called a demonstration effect.

That people who participate directly in activities have their consciousness raised, or their morale affected – for better or for worse – is fairly indisputable. It is a difficult methodological problem to establish how far people feel 'involved' as onlookers on a scenario when they have no direct role or stake. To test this theory is beyond the sensitivity of conventional sociological method. However, it concerns a minor point of theory and is not such an important task as explicating the broader theoretical point that organisations and activities in general affect a neighbourhood. This is to say that not only are direct participants affected by such activity but that it affects a far more generalised sector of the population.

This seems to present an extremely important point of theory for community work to resolve. There seem to be two foci to a community worker's effects in a theoretical sense. First, a great deal of the effect of organisation introduced into a small area relates to the relatively small group of individuals who are most centrally involved. They absorb much of the community worker's attention, and the results they present in terms of increased skills, know-how and self-confidence are tangible evidence to the worker of a project's effectiveness. The second effect – on the wider population – is more difficult to assess. If it is posed in terms of improved service delivery, this is relatively straightforward. However, community work theory on the subject goes beyond this. It suggests an 'area effect' which may be expressed in one of two popular forms: either a raising of the quality of life in the area, or a raising of consciousness – very often meant as political awareness.

It is not really contentious to suggest that an improved range of services bring an improved quality of life, if that is the measure of 'quality of life'. The wider ambitions above may sound less convincing. However, there is room for dispute in both these types of proposition. Individual services may affect tiny proportions of a population, for example playgroups and advice centres. Thus area-effect may be a less direct effect of such community work than imagined. Yet the knowledge of the services' existence and an awareness of the activity going on in a community without actually using or organising them could have quite a strong influence on people's satisfaction with living in the area, and given a level of publicised political activity, greatly affect their attitudes to local authority affairs and their role as local citizens.

The various strands of this argument are not new to community workers. The reason for presenting them in this form is to stress that they do hold a series of testable propositions. The more subtle effects proposed in such a theory present difficult research problems. This may be a deterrent to community workers whose resources are already short and whose expertise lies elsewhere. However, it does underline an area where community work's theories are relatively unsubstantiated by hard evidence. In the long term – or sooner if one is to note the alacrity with which some boroughs have recently cut their community work teams – resources must be found to undertake empirical testing as a guide to the direction of workers' own efforts and to lay a better-argued claim for resources for community work as a desirable service. It may represent an issue to community workers regarding the prominence in their theories of educational effort towards individuals or neighbours.

There is a point of tension in policy theory which needs to be considered under this section. The argument that community work can be a means to improve the quality of life – as discussed above – has appeared in some policy documents such as the Seebohm Report (1968), often accompanied by the notion that community work can be a means of reducing the incidence of conventional social problems at the local level. This involves a policy argument, as to whether or not community work should be conceived in this way, which has caused tension in some local authorities between social workers and community workers. There is also a practice argument involved as to whether or not community work can and does affect an area in such a fashion.

There are simple answers – that, for example, playgroups ease the pressure on childminding and nursery facilities, and squatting associations ease certain kinds of pressure on housing resources. There are also more generalised effects, such as reports from one police authority that a summer play scheme resulted in the first ever reduction in summer-holiday vandalism. These propositions are not the same, however, as one which says a raising of morale and increased satisfaction and 'identity' with an area reduce the tendency to deviance and distress. Community work projects are often so small as to make the likelihood of measurable effects of this sort somewhat unreasonable to expect. The principle, however, appears basically sound and improved documentation in suitable project areas could increase our knowledge on the subject.

A far more likely area for the development of such a theory relates to the people with whom the community worker directly works rather than the huge populations in which he or she is often based. Young and Wilmott (1962) and many writers afterwards have emphasised the good neighbourliness of working-class communities. Community workers develop organisations for service or political purposes, yet in encouraging individuals to local prominence they may be developing neighbourliness of a very powerful sort. Preliminary interviews by this writer with leaders of local action groups have shown that their involvement in giving personal help to neighbours had increased enormously. Moreover, the aid and advice given included a huge range of subjects normally falling within the province of the statutory services. Quality of care may clearly be at issue here, but preliminary care and referral are potentially a valuable service to existing agencies. This is a relatively undocumented aspect of community work. Increased attention to this phenomenon in research terms would, it seems, greatly strengthen community work's claim for statutory support.

The Question of Role

Theory of a different type is involved in one of the traditional areas of debate in community work. This was discussed at length by earlier writers such as Batten (1967) and Goetschius (1968), and involves the 'non-directive' versus 'directive' approaches. This does not involve sociological ideas such as those in the former theories discussed, but a type of learning theory belonging more to the discipline of educational psychology. It is, in these terms, technically beyond the present writer to assess which is the more effective method of intervention. In any event, the theoretical question seems to have been superseded by ethical concerns. What was once seen as non-interfering and respectful may now be seen as irresponsible. For example, a participant in a recent community work conference related that he had accompanied a local committee member to a meeting with local government officials. When this person had 'dried up' in the intimidating environment of formality and officialdom the worker did not know whether it was correct or not to intervene. This may show that the issue is not yet dead, but the scant sympathy shown for the worker's dilemma illustrated the change of attitude on such issues in recent years. Probably the issue has not so much disappeared as become more sophisticated. The dignity accrued to the recipient in the non-directive method is doubtless still important yet the principle of subsuming the 'clients' ' tangible needs to the workers' process goals is, hopefully, disappearing.

Women in Community Work

Certain issues of practice theory overlap with theoretical issues discussed in other categories above. For example, the role performed by women in community development activity may be illuminated by a better understanding of contextual theory, that is the extent to which culture affects a woman's predisposition to act and in what way. It may also be affected by a social policy theory; if woman is the custodian of the 'sphere of reproduction' and this is the focus of community work's efforts then she assumes potentially an extremely important role. In any event, the experience of day-to-day practice has shown female responses in the community work situation to have distinctive characteristics. Contrary to the dismissiveness of political sociology – that woman is conservative and deferential to the political views of her husband – she has been shown in a variety of local confrontations to be more radical, tougher, more persistent and less easily browbeaten than her male neighbours. One book in particular has helped to assemble knowledge on the subject (Mayo, 1977) and many individual cases have been reported where women had taken the initiative collectively – notably from Northern Ireland. Certainly this is an area of knowledge that has to be more systematically appraised and absorbed into the practice theory of the profession.

Tenants' Associations

The point alluded to above, that one analysis of community work's role directs it to working-class organisation based on housing, involves a theoretical point which is slightly at variance with the evidence. Women do not appear more frequently as the leading lights of tenants' associations – which represent the chief protagonists of working-class interests in this respect at the local level. Possibly this is because these tend to be long-standing organisations, and women are less disposed or enabled to take part in them. Certainly many reported instances of all-female action have been of a short-term and issue-centred nature.

Tenants' associations possibly represent the most persistent feature of community development in this country – with the exception of community associations which have less significance theoretically. They flourish despite the setbacks following the Housing Finance Act of 1972, and tend to figure high in the priorities of individual community workers' programmes of work. They may be regarded as representing tenants' most important material interest following the wage packet.

The extent to which this is the case, or to which the tenants' association is regarded as the appropriate means to protect such interests, could be better illustrated by research. There is the phenomenon, for example, that those most secure in their housing rights frequently become the leaders of tenants' associations and then show little sophistication in regarding housing as a right when it is, in fact, the rights of others which are at issue. Moreover, many tenants may not see such an organisation as altogether politically legitimate. Tenants' associations offer probably the best single opportunity to the community worker. A more consistent attempt to integrate them into a policy theory – with the benefit of increased empirical evidence – could greatly help in the evaluation of such work.

The Unattached Worker

A point of theory – arising out of model building – has appeared as an issue in community work practice, though this may be more real as an analytic than as a practical phenomenon. An earlier, popular model of the community worker presented him or her as an unattached worker – a roving catalyst to community activity with no well-defined brief or clearly categorised expertise. This somewhat romantic role is now regarded uneasily among community workers who increasingly seem to seek a tangible base for their activities. This may take the form of a resource centre, advice centre, or one of the many other local facilities which have been the subject of experiments in recent years. There is, however, hint of another preference which may be regarded as an aspect of the same trend, namely to adopt a clearer professional identity in conventional terms. Individual planners and solicitors based in law centres are examples of professionals who have made enormous contributions to community work. This, and unsatisfactory experience with the simple, 'unattached worker' label, has encouraged some workers to acquire conventional practical qualifications. One meets community workers taking housing management qualifications or becoming specialists in planning law, and the trend is encouraged by Thomas (1978) who presents a persuasive case for assuming the identity of social planner.

Allied to the model of professional roles at issue here, there is involved – though not very prominently – a question of practice theory. It is not clear how effectiveness varies in degree or kind between the 'unattached' approach and a local community work strategy based on a tangible project – for example with a 'shop front' feature – but it is a theoretical question to bear in mind. Community workers seldom have much choice between strategies due to the low level of resources made available to their projects, but case records in time may show one differentially effective *vis-à-vis* the other. In any event, the accumulation of evidence on the matter can only be to the benefit of practice theory.

The Community Worker as Educator

Additional to this issue arising from model building is another involved in the preference by some practitioners and writers – including the present one – for classifying the community worker as an educator. The debate on community work as part of or separate from social work contains at least as much polemic as sound argument, and the reliance of community workers on social services departments for their main employment does not enhance the purity of the analysis. None the less, many, in private discussion, appear to prefer the 'education' label and a shift in practice theory might be implied by this trend.

Compensatory education is the term to describe a process of redressing imbalance of social-cum-political skills in an adult population which, simply, is what community work in these terms is about. It may be argued that the issues faced by adults – housing, jobs, the environment – are the *raison d'être* of community work and the task is therefore defined as one involving the adult population. However, there are deep-seated attitudinal factors lying behind these problems which are a function of life-long experience rather than day-to-day issues (Tasker, 1978). Dealing with these may not be best accomplished by a process of compensatory education, rather by an educational effort directed towards earlier stages of individuals' experience. In short, the community worker as educator may have to seriously consider the way that children and young people fit into his or her strategy.

One development in recent years appears conducive to this trend. Adventure playleaders have increasingly accepted a community dimension to their work, whereas formerly they protected the right of kids to play for its own sake and resisted the political orientation of community workers. The *de facto* involvement of playgrounds in some local education authority plans and the race issue which has manifested itself on some playgrounds has possibly been responsible for playleaders taking a broader view of their work. Direct attempts to introduce democratic training into play may be due more to the influence of community work or an aspect of the absorption of community work ideas in the helping professions generally (see Chapter 11 by Brian Munday for a further discussion of this point). This is one indication at least that the tie-up between young people and community work may become practically and theoretically closer.

The Concept of Need

A supposedly operational concept in earlier community work is due for reconsideration. 'Self-defined need' was current in the helping professions in an earlier period and absorbed in community work. It was supposed to inform the way a worker set his priorities and seemed closely allied to the concept of the 'unattached worker' mentioned above. That 'community needs' and preferences do not 'emerge' or express themselves so magically has surely been realised by fieldworkers. The more random fact finding and opinion sounding based on pure leg-work by the community worker has an indispensable place, but it is not an adequate strategy in itself to discover the state of need and opinion in a locality. In summary, the skills and sensitivity of a fieldworker are not alone adequate to deal with this aspect of practice. To be succesful it also needs planning and a systematic input of information.

This is an incomplete summary of theoretical issues in practice, but the observations suggest two major issues in the way community work methods have developed. First, there is a need to reflect upon the concepts involved in a given piece of field strategy, to order these and recognise that they involve theoretical propositions. The second point is that while more articulate theorising may make the questions clearer, the answers to questions often lie in more thorough assembling of information.

Community workers cannot be their own field researchers to any great extent but they can become data-oriented. Nor should they simply be ideologues. Ideology is unavoidable and vital, but cannot build a good, accreditable code of practice on its own. To do this it is necessary for community workers to become at least as good theorisers as they are ideologists – remembering that currently the balance of these is often the other way round.

CONCLUSIONS

The most important thing to recognise in assessing the state of theory in community work is that community work is about class. The efforts of community workers are concerned with certain kinds of underprivilege among working-class people which are, in turn, related to the more familiar types discussed in the welfare literature. Tackling lack of organisational capability is not really possible so long as there is insufficient understanding by professional workers of the rest of the culture in which they are working, into which they are trying to introduce new skills and attitudes, and from which they are trying to encourage particular kinds of initiatives. Conventional sociology has not really been adequate to the task of providing this type of intervention with the knowledge it requires, so that an understanding of cultural context and its reaction to various aspects of practice is perhaps the greatest need in the theoretical development of the profession.

Community work's internal research efforts should not be applied here as the subject matter is basically sociological in nature and a research structure exists within sociology which should be able to respond to such professional demands. Closely related to this is the need to develop a greater understanding of practice methods, effects and effectiveness. The questions surrounding these can be generalised, as in the comparison mentioned above about issue-centred or ongoing organisations, or can relate to comparisons of particular kinds of project such as advice centres, resource centres, newspapers, playgrounds or the many other kinds of project-base for community work. A successful understanding of these will not be achieved until research resources are brought into community work. Leaving social context to be studied by sociologists is inevitable, but community work will not advance satisfactorily without monitoring and assessing its own methods.

A methodology must be developed for recording reactions to and indications of social change, to establish paradigms for measurement, and scales of comparison. Research methodology, however, is not the main obstacle, rather research resources. Since the Home Office Community Development Projects there has not been a co-ordinated plan for community work to sustain research activity on the scale required. Realisation of the importance of research on this type of intervention is necessary at central government and local government levels likewise.

Community workers, too, must make their efforts to convince independent funding authorities of the need for monitoring and researching and have it built into community work programmes, as in the case of the Young Volunteer Force project in Stoke (Key *et al*, 1976). They may be confident of the productivity of their work, but more data could add to their ability to convince sponsors and improve community work's credibility overall.

Community work, if seen as an aspect of the working-class movement, needs the relationship to other sections of this movement clarified, and the support of empirical evidence for the theory of change involved. Working-class consciousness and self-reliance may be raised through various kinds of community work activity – it is certainly intended to be – but its most effective forms in relation to the general effects of the Labour movement need better information. The clearest link theoretically may be the support given by community work to tenants' associations. Many indeed argue that housing should be the second basis of organised effort in achieving working-class emancipation. There is also the question of the relationship to the women's movement, which may be just as important a question for community work.

If the priority for theorising in community work can possibly be unravelled it lies probably in the area of contextual theory and practice. An increased knowledge of the communities in which they are working plus better information systems in respect of specific actions would enable community workers better to understand their methods in relation to the dynamics of the culture concerned. This implies a dynamically oriented sociology. Further, it implies monitoring.

As an activity, theorising has not been popular in community work.

Its stimulus seems to have other origins – some mentioned above. 'Cause-and-effect' does not stand out as the main rationale for the job. In fact it does not appear to be empirical factors at all which were originally behind the development of the practice; rather various kinds of ideological impetus such as Christianity, Liberalism, Marxism, bourgeois humanitarianism, and ideals and principles from a variety of other helping professions. One might adapt Radford's slogan: 'Don't agonise – theorise!' (1978).

Community work, in as much as it is salaried and to an extent professionalised, cannot survive in the current climate of welfare politics when based mainly on well-meaning individual inclination and popular liberal ideals. Its claims must be supported with good theory based on evidence collected as systematically as methodology and resources allow. To do this practitioners must become theory-minded, and attract resources into community work to carry out research to enable its claims to be established as irrefutably as possible.

REFERENCES

Alinsky, S. D. (1969). *Reveille for Radicals* (New York: Random House).

Batten, T. R. (1967). *The Non-Directive Approach in Group and Community Work* (London: OUP).

Benington, J. (1974). 'Strategies for change at the local level: some reflections', in D. Jones and M. Mayo (eds) *Community Work: One* (London: Routledge).

Bryant, R. (1972). 'Community action', *British Journal of Social Work*, vol. 2, no. 2.

Central Council for Education and Training in Social Work (1978). 'Issues relating to one-year postgraduate CQSW courses' (mimeo) (London: CCETSW).

Cockburn, C. (1977). *The Local State* (London: Pluto).

Goetschius, G. (1968). *Working with Community Groups* (London: Routledge).

Gulbenkian Foundation (1968). *Community Work and Social Change – A Report on Training* (London: Longmans).

Hoggart, R. (1957). *The Uses of Literacy* (London: Chatto and Windus).

Hoyland, J. (1976). *Community Festivals Handbook* (London: YVFF).

Key, M. *et al.* (1976). *Evaluation Theory and Community Work* (London: YVFF).

Klein, J. (1963). *Working with Groups* (London: Hutchinson).

Leissner, A. (1975). 'Models for community workers and community youth workers', *Social Work Today*, vol. 5, no. 22 (February).

Mayo, M. (1975). 'Community development: a radical alternative?', in R. Bailey and M. Brake (eds) *Radical Social Work* (London: Arnold).

Mayo, M. (ed.) (1977). *Women in the Community* (London: Routledge).

National Community Development Project (1975). *Forward plan 1975–6* (London: CDP Information and Intelligence Unit).

Newcomb, T. M. (1943). *Personality and Social Change* (New York: Holt).
Norris, M. (1977). 'A formula for identifying styles of community work', *Community Development Journal*, vol. 12, no. 1.
Radford, J. (1978). 'Don't agonise – organise!', in P. Curno (ed.), *Political Issues and Community Work* (London: Routledge).
Reid, I. (1977). *Social Class Differences in Britain* (London: Open Books).
Rothman, J. (1974), 'Three models of community organisation practice', in F. M. Cox *et al.* (eds), *Strategies of Community Organisation* Itasca, Ill.: Peacock).
Seebohm Report: (1968). *Report of the Committee on Local Authority and Allied Personal Social Services* (London: HMSO).
Tasker, L. (1978). 'Class, culture and community work', in P. Curno (ed.) *Political Issues and Community Work* (London: Routledge).
Thomas, D. N. (1975). 'Said Alice, "The great question certainly was, what?" ', *Social Work Today* (27 November).
Thomas, D. N. (1978). 'Community work, social change and social planning', in P. Curno (ed.), *Political Issues and Community Work* (London: Routledge).
Young, M. and Willmott, P. (1962). *Family and Kinship in East London* (Harmondsworth: Penguin).
Ziblatt, D. (1963). 'High school extra-curricular activities and political socialisation', *Annals of American Academy of Political Science.*

Chapter 3

MAKING SENSE OF THEORY

Jalna Hanmer and Hilary Rose

This chapter reviews the dominant theoretical approaches to community work and relates them to the socio-economic circumstances which surround their origins. Our general perspective views community work, such as social work, town planning, and social policy (indeed, the welfare state itself), as neither a purely technical matter, nor as one containing any built-in guarantees as to its controlling or liberatory nature. We both share and acknowledge the hunch of many community workers that they work in a country where Catch 22 rules; that after a long, complex and exhausting community struggle when victory looks as if it is coming into view (a motorway has been nearly blocked, the local authority is almost certainly not going to close the battered women's refuge), the community worker's feelings often border on paranoia. Do 'they' want the motorway blocked as the state becomes less willing to spend money on the urban infrastructure, have 'we' just helped the local state evade its responsibilities and co-opt a social movement?

These difficult and serious questions have no easy answers given the increasing theoretical and practical sophistication of community workers. The occupational group having 'discovered' community work in the heady days of the mid-1960s and early 1970s, where theory was joyfully abandoned and practice embraced, now finds itself in a difficult world, where welfare is under siege and where the condition of the people they seek to serve slowly but steadily deteriorates. In this context, the old *élan* of a group which believed that it was destined to act as a catalyst to bring about significant and far-reaching social change is worn into a more critical and self-sceptical mould.

These sharp contradictions in which community work finds itself at the end of the 1970s serve to stimulate interest both in present theoretical issues and also in a re-examination of the roots of community work itself. Although such a survey as we make in this chapter is inevitably synoptic, we begin with what we characterise as the colonial inheritance of the community development tradition, then move to a discussion of three competing paradigms of community work: the consensual, the pluralist, and structural versions of conflict theory. Within these three conceptions of community work theory and practice lies a growing feminist concern. The analysis we make here is enriched by the wealth of both the practice and the theories developed by the women's liberation movement, and draws both on our joint empirical work in the London Borough of Islington and on work carried out by our students in London and Bradford.

THE COLONIAL INHERITANCE

Community work in Britain is embedded in the history of colonialism. Leaper (1968) as a conservative writer and Mayo (1975) as a Marxist jointly point to the long history of the concept and practice of 'community development' as it was first termed, in the context of British West Africa. Initially, and some of us observing the wheel making a full turn may be forgiven an ironic moment at the discovery with Freire (1972) of community adult education, community development was then seen specifically as an education activity. Thus *Education Policy in British Tropical Africa* (Colonial Office, 1925) represents a pioneering text. *Mass Education in African Society* (Colonial Office, 1935) published ten years later, continues to reflect that contradiction between the needs of the colonialists simultaneously to maintain social control and to advance a people moving toward de-colonisation in the context of a deteriorating political situation in Europe (with war threatening), and the rising expectations of an agrarian people who wished for an end of exploitation, subordinate status and poverty. With the break-up of empire in the Second World War, and its aftermath, community development became *the* path of social development, favoured by the British Colonial Office and the countries that made up the United Nations alike.

Retrospectively, it is easy to understand the convergence of the two. The United Nations, for all its commitment to a post-colonial world, was yet to experience the advent of the new black African and Arab states. For a while, even where an indigenous leadership had replaced a colonial administration, de-colonisation by agreement was a very different political experience to de-colonisation through struggle and even bloody war. Against 'community development' with its thesis of consensual development were to be set the writings of Frantz Fanon, who argued that internationalisation of the specific form of colonial oppression could only be destroyed through the violent struggle of the oppressed against the oppressors (Fanon, 1968).

Nevertheless, in the late 1950s there was agreement – even consensus: 'Community development is a movement designed to create better living for the whole community, with the active participation and on the initiative of the local community' (Colonial Office, 1958). Even in 1968, a year marked by the Tet offensive as the most dramatic moment of struggle by the Vietnamese people against a neo-imperialist army of occupation, the United Nations continued to attempt to maintain the thesis of change through consensus: 'The people themselves are united with the governmental authorities . . . Two essential elements, the participation of the people themselves in an effort to improve their level of living with as much reliance as possible on their own initiative, and the provision of technical and other services in ways that encourage initiative and self-help' (cited Leaper, 1968). Community development, this concept fashioned by the Colonial Office, and adopted by the first phase of post-colonial governments in the United Nations, emphasised the common interests of those living within a specific geographical locality. Concepts of class and imperialism with their conflictual bases of solidarity were laid to one side in order to perpetuate those concepts and theories which suggested more manageable forms of solidarity.

Within this view of community development lay the shadow of the classical nineteenth-century longing for the regeneration of *Gemeinschaft* within the atomic social relations of capitalism. The settlement movement discussed in more detail in Chapter 1 by Peter Baldock was the concrete expression of this desire to recreate the social relations of the village within the urban slum. The new squirearchy were those young men and women from the upper echelons of society who volunteered to live in the settlements, who by their example and their humanity were to help gentle those that the Victorians feared as the dangerous classes. It was this consensual model recreating community in neighbourhoods, which as Mayo (1975) has reminded us, was perpetuated within the tradition of neighbourhood work as integral to community development.

COMMUNITY DEVELOPMENT AT HOME

It was thus appropriate after the war that the London Council of Social Service opened a community development section. In the 1950s Muriel Smith, who was subsequently to play a significant part within the next two decades of community work, as for example a key worker in the central group of the CDP, sought to initiate community associations on the new council housing estates. On meeting with local tenants she found that some estates had formed local tenants' groups to promote neighbourliness by providing varying activities for residents. These new groups were responding to the need created by large-scale rehousing of people. Familes and households were seeking to resettle themselves in a new environment that often had changed in three major ways: in terms of place, people, and physical structures. A move of even a quarter of a mile could be felt as major, new neighbours replaced the old, and two-storey terraces opening on to a street were exchanged for medium and tower blocks fitted into landscaped common areas of grass and paths. These changes curtailed access to the life of the community, creating unwanted isolation while at the same time within the home the often poor soundproofing reduced desired privacy, thus fuelling the need to negotiate with neighbours.

Muriel Smith realised these new groups were more appropriate to the needs of the new estates than the community association form of organisation, and began to help them with what they saw as their problems. She was joined by Ilys Booker, and the basis for what has become the London Association of Housing Estates began to take shape. George Goetschius documented the growth of their organisation; the aims and method of work corresponded to aims and dominant ideas about community development (or community organisation, as it was termed in the USA and taught in schools of social work) (Goetschius, 1969). While the fashions in community work were to diversify, it is important to realise that this method fitted this social situation neatly.

In antagonism to this officially approved grouping was set the Association of Tenants and Residents, substantially influenced by Communist militants. Its peak was the St Pancras rent strike (Moorhouse *et al.*, 1972), but it none the less had great difficulties in maintaining an active membership.

Ilys Booker (and it is interesting how far the shifts in approaches can be matched by the movements of particular individuals), went on to work for a family-centred project in Notting Hill (Mitton and Morrison, 1972). As we shall describe later on, Notting Hill was also the test bed for the ideas of the New Left. The Notting Hill Family Project was the inspiration of Pearl Jephcott and had a star-studded management committee, including Eileen Younghusband. The project was tied to the settlement house tradition. The focus throughout the life of the project was on autonomous local groups with the aim of lifting themselves out of the quagmire of inner-city deprivation. When later T. R. Batten, who had worked on community development in West Africa and had developed the first course for community workers in Britain at the Institute of Education during the 1950s for workers from colonial and ex-colonial countries, joined the management committee, a dispute arose centring on the use of resources. He saw the project as an opportunity to test ideas developed in colonial countries and he argued that resources should be used only to further the worker's function and not for technical aids such as specialised workers, premises, equipment. The bootstrap effort should be total.

Ilys Booker's illness during the project, and death before its completion, was experienced as a great loss, but none the less the project was seen as the definitive test of the applicability of both the colonial tradition of community development and the traditional concept of 'community' in Britain. This study was to symbolise both at home and abroad that for community work to be successful in the future it must consist of a combination of governmental aid and local initiative.

THE GROWTH OF THE WELFARE STATE

While this influence within the subsequent history of community work is a matter of interest to those directly involved in the theory and practice of community work, it, like other influences, becomes of much broader significance set into the context of the dramatic expansion of the welfare state between the 1940s and 1970s. Whilst in qualitative terms social policy analysts had written of the growth of the welfare state, few had drawn attention to the overall size of the social service budget, and its changed relationship to GNP. To some extent, it is arguable that the liberal ideology within which the discussion of both social policy and social and community work were set during those years, had served to defend and extend welfare. One might even say that the liberal ideologues had actually been a little reticent over the price of the bill. For our purposes, it is important to stress the sheer scale of welfare within the economy. Where, in the 1920s a mere 4 per cent of GNP was spent on social services, at the eve of war it stood at 11 per cent, and by 1975 social services took no less than 25 per cent of GNP (Gough, 1975). Initially, economic commentators tended to note the shift in a postwar Britain from a manufacturing to a service economy. What these figures serve to highlight is a shift towards a public service economy and with it the expansion of the social service occupations. With this expansion was to come what Wilensky (1964) termed 'The professionalization of everyone'.

Amongst these newly developed professional groups were the social workers. Community work was much slower in its growth. By the time it made its appearance upon the scene it was no longer possible to embrace the professional path with the same kind of confidence which had accompanied the development of social work. Eileen Younghusband was paradoxically to foster both, using the 1947 Carnegie Trust Report as her trojan horse to introduce social casework into the university in general and the London School of Economics in particular in 1954, and then the Gulbenkian Report (Gulbenkian Foundation, 1968) to recreate the strategy for community work in the 1960s. However, whilst social work developed via

Younghusband (1959) and Seebohm (1968) towards professional power to become the object of external critique, most memorably first by Wootton (1959) and then Sinfield (1969), and subsequently through auto-critique by radical social work in the magazine *Casecon* or the Bailey and Brake (1975) edited collection of essays, community work's slower start meant that by the time the occupation had arrived in sufficient numerical terms, the high tide of professionalism had passed. Instead the community workers found themselves trapped in a contradiction where they both sought to control the training and define the task just like any other professionalising group, while using the rhetoric and even promoting the reality of the claims of deprofessionalisation (Lonsdale, 1975; Cox and Derricourt, 1975).

But while the Association of Community Workers were to debate professionalisation and deprofessionalisation, no such crisis in values was experienced by the Gulbenkian Committee which began the campaign to include community work education and training in professional social work courses, initially focusing on LSE. The oldest social work course in the country, with a deeply entrenched psychoanalytic model, became the battleground for what was to be subsequently termed the unitary approach. Unlike Britain, the American model of social work included case, group and community work, and the American-trained George Goetschius, as the first lecturer in community work at LSE, formed the spearhead of the attack. The problems encountered are carefully documented in *Community Work Two* and were experienced at least in part by other courses as the initiative to broaden existing social work education was taken up elsewhere (Jones and Mayo, 1975).

How to broaden social work education was initially unclear. Were there to be community work options on courses as in the American model? Was there some way of presenting a more integrated model for social work, one that would allow for workers with individuals to have a richer base from which to assess and help the client while community work training took place elsewhere? New writing on the relationship between case, group and community work began to appear in 1973 and seemed to offer a way out of the dilemmas created by traditional teaching of social casework (Pincus and Minahan, 1973; Goldstein, 1973). While some community workers attack the spread of the unitary approach on social work courses as an example of welfare imperialism, it needs to be recognised that the form of individual work carried out by caseworkers was being transformed by reorganisation of social work services (Armstrong and Gill, 1978; Ley, 1978). In the new Seebohm departments, psychoanalytic casework was more often than not inappropriate. New models for individual work had to be found; ones not so dependent on psychopathology as explanation in order that the economic and general cultural needs of individuals could be recognised and included in the assessment so that appropriate help could be offered.

The growing occupational group of community workers found employment within the burgeoning welfare state, working either directly for central or local government or for that complex of semi-official to entirely voluntary agencies which were developed during the latter 1960s. Social casework's reputation had been tarnished by the charge that it was too tied into social control through its pre-occupation with the client's psychopathology at the expense of helping with the client's problems. Community work with its assumption of the normality of the people it worked with offered a fresh approach (Goetschius, 1969).

The rediscovery of poverty during the 1960s with the official understanding that it was limited to specific "pockets of poverty" (a view which conflicted with the evidence but which none the less captured the political imagination), led to a belief that poverty was to be found located in specific limited geographical areas. The policy response was to set in train a series of spatially based strategies against poverty. Beginning with Education Priority Areas, extending through the Community Development Project, the Six Cities Project, Housing Action Areas, Comprehensive Community Planning, by the mid-1970s inner-city programme followed inner-city programme. What is important to us here is that many of these programmes, which echoed in albeit suitably muted form the enthusiasm for public participation of the American War on Poverty, required community workers for their implementation. Nor was the voluntary sector to be outdone; it sponsored projects and began to interest itself in the question of the task and training of community workers. Central within this activity was the prestigious committee, noted earlier, sponsored by the Gulbenkian Foundation and chaired by Eileen Younghusband. The first report (Gulbenkian Foundation, 1968) drew attention to three areas of intervention: community development, community organisation, and social planning. While their first report recognised the consensual model it was not until the report of the second committee (Gulbenkian Foundation, 1973), that community action was mentioned and a pluralistic conflict model was publicly acknowledged within the discussions of this key grouping.

Retrospectively, it would be not unfair to argue that the community development model maintained its hegemony over community work theory and practice throughout the 1950s and surprisingly far into the 1960s, but that the growth of the welfare state and those problems spoken of in shorthand as 'the rediscovery of poverty' revealed the inadequacies of the model in these new circumstances. From liberal and social democratic political theory, a pluralist model of conflict was introduced to tackle the problems of poverty and social antagonisms which had emerged during the 1960s.

At the same moment, from the New Left movement of the 1960s which embraced libertarians, Marxists, black groups and the nascent women's liberation movement, came a tumult of competing but predominantly structurally based theories of social change through conflict. Thus the late 1960s ushered in a new period of competing paradigms in community work. Community development remained and remains influential but was increasingly jostled by the new theorists of pluralistic and structural conflict. It is to this present situation of competing paradigms that we now turn.

PLURALISTS

It is difficult to discuss pluralist models of community work separately from the structural, as much of what now can be labelled pluralist began in antagonism to the old consensual model of community development. The differences which were subsequently to be visible were initially obscure both to participants and observers. At one extreme, community is conceived of as a unified social system consisting of family, neighbourhood and friends, the *Gemeinschaft* of F. Tonnies and the traditional society of academic sociologists where, as we have been discussing, social action and control flow from a common identity of interests. Tonnies conceived the opposite type of society to be based on the chillier relationships of association, secondary social contacts that fragment social life, but it was left to Marx to map out the true opposite: a community divided over the production of wealth where class was pitted against class in a relentless struggle of antithetical interests. In between lies the pluralist thesis of conflict where the differential, but not antithetical, interests of citizens leads to institutionalised conflict.

This conflict, however, gives rise to consensus not revolution, and is well illustrated by the abrasive quality of Alinsky-style community work (1969 and 1972). This seemed to offer the possibility of people themselves through collective action bringing about the far-reaching changes that community development and social casework had denied; yet stability through continuous change may occur because there are no zero sum games, where one person's gain is another's loss. The image in this model is of Alinsky on a white horse leading a smash-and-grab raid on the town hall for a share of the unlimited goodies. In a more realistic model of pluralism, particularly following recent cuts in public expenditure, it is accepted that resources are limited and zero sum games the order of the day. To generate consensus from continual conflict where there are real losers requires more sophisticated strategies. Participation, the one unlimited resource, theoretically has much to offer (Rose, 1976). Tokenistic, or pseudo-participation, misses the point as citizen alienation may be increased by attempts to cool people into decisions taken in advance, or where only small relatively unimportant aspects are open to negotiation and change (Arnstein, 1969). A fully active society, one based on a cybernetic model (Rose and Hanmer, 1975), needs decision-making organisational structures where decision-making and planning units are less segregated than at present. A scheme devised by the American sociologist Amitai Etzioni calls for initial plans which provide a context where planners and those to be affected by the decisions work together to complete them (Etzioni, 1968). His concept of the 'conflict-limiting capsule' was taken up by David Donnison and applied to the local state in Britain (Donnison, 1973). The mini-town hall (or conflict-limiting capsule), is a blueprint for an organisation with enough latitude to allow the details of 'who gets what when' to be worked out collectively. Donnison argues that significant citizen participation will allow endless subdivision and reallocation of welfare resources and through the efficient harnessing of participation zero sum games can be avoided. In practice, however, these visions have not been tried out in full and experience other problems when partially applied. Witness Cynthia Cockburn's analysis of how one such capsule, a local authority-sponsored neighbourhood council, worked in practice (Cockburn, 1977).

Cockburn sets out how the state and capital can benefit from and exploit and disarm progressive ideas and people. She points sensitively to the situation of the community worker, whose subjective consciousness sees structural antagonism, and who believes that the actions of the community groups he or she works with will lead to significant change, but may none the less objectively serve to shore up the inadequacies of the local state. In her discussion of the conflict model she describes how central government through various special projects and financial schemes encouraged local government to engage in participatory exercises, to promote events that exposed the local state to criticism and change.

Managing the local state is problematic in many ways. As Cockburn's study illustrates, people participate differentially, which affects the upward flow of information while the downward flow, the response to local authority initiatives and ideas, may not be positive. Complex structures require sophisticated management. Community work becomes a new way of trouble-shooting; in cybernetic theory it is the feedback loop that corrects system imbalance. A fully active model of society requires active participation by all its citizens, information dissemination and processing on an extensive scale, ample opportunities for discussion and conflict, and organisational forms whose structures have sealed the larger questions from debate, but within which scope exists for minor, but sufficient, variations to construct social consensus. But as all community workers know, it is far from easy for the local state to promote its conception of appropriate participation among the associations, neighbourhoods and families that constitute its population.

The central state can be seen to have similar problems in managing the local. Central government does not always have the control over local authorities it would like. Positive incentives are used; but these do not work effectively with local authorities who cannot be enticed, or who cannot understand how, to apply for the various and changing grant programmes. They do not all have managers who like deficit spending, bargain basement offers and clever accounting. Negative sanctions are equally problematic, whether legislative or financial; witness the continuing resistance of some local authorities to comprehensive education. At the very least constant negotiation is required.

The dramatic growth of the scale and range of the state's intervention in social welfare laid the foundation for the re-emergence of community work and community politics, both the consensual community development and the conflictual community action variants. Individuals may be motivated by a feeling that community is being lost. Conservative theorists such as Nisbet make a curious unstated alliance with Bethnal Green sociology, mourning the loss of working-class community in the face of urban redevelopment and change (Nisbet, 1967). Where Bethnal Green sociology suggests that a community could be maintained through more sensitive social planning (Young and Willmott, 1957), Nisbet argues that the growth of the desire for community has occurred because the state is extending itself at the expense of the intermediate associations of family, neighbourhood, and the various voluntary asociations of a locality. The type of relationships that make up the state is said to sap the vitality of these intermediate associations and threatens to destroy them. Certainly the state has become more pervasive in the recent past. Margaret Stacey's two studies of the small market town of Banbury illustrate the extent to which the national state has increasingly penetrated the local level, while the local state has increasingly extended its activities (Stacey, 1960; Stacey, *et al.*, 1975).

The state offers a particular type of relationship between individuals and groups, and this may be genuinely found wanting. Struggles against the local (and national) state can have an element of opposition to inhumanity – to relationships devoid of proper respect, feeling, response. There is a sense in which local (and national) struggles are crusades for recognition of the humanness of those who protest. It is no surprise that the new wave of paid community work in Britain began with people dislocated from their familiar neighbourhoods by rebuilding and slum clearance.

Consensual community development was followed by more conflictual models as the focus of discontent around housing shifted from problems of resettlement to problems of the loss of a home through particularly vicious forms of slum landlordism. Islington became the target of a pace-setting campaign to force the local authority to take a more active role by compulsory purchase of the speculator's property. Anne Power (1973) describes the battle of Stonefield Street where the local authority, not expecting a positive reply, finally agreed to ask the Minister of Housing to act. This strategy was resisted by those groups that analysed the local state as the enemy, but once the objective was achieved the local authority became an ally and, by this route, community politics as a form of revolutionary struggle became those of reform. An analysis based on antithetical class interests gave way to a pluralist conception of the state.

Nor was the initiative left solely in the hands of the community groups. Local authorities, such as Islington, which understood that modern corporate management required high-quality information, were quick to recognise the significance of community participation as crucial to managerial success. While other authorities, whose councillors were less drawn from the new managerial and technical classes, remained loyal to dirigistic forms of government, Islington pioneered participation as a new approach of managing the local state. A string of participatory forms were devised by a special committee with information services, financial and other material resources to dispense to local groups engaged in one-off exercises in upward and downward information flows, to substantially funded experimental neighbourhood forums to consolidate and extend local voluntary efforts. To characterise the approach as pluralist is to simplify and even hide the multiplicity of ways that conflicts of interest can be conceptualised and played out.

None the less, the ultimate importance of the support of the council remains a central feature, whether for the compulsory purchase of a large privately owned estate or for much less ambitious community group goals. The struggle by the tenants of the New River Estate in Islington was punctilious in its efforts to avoid encapsulation, using tactics to maintain its autonomy ranging from producing their own minutes of joint meetings with the local authority to never using local authority premises for their meetings. Less idealistic strategies were also pursued. Others, having begun by challenging the local councillors through community groups, concluded by replacing councillors by themselves. Volunteering for personal co-option added a new dimension to the theory of the active society. Leading activists pioneered the way for the institutionalisation of conflict through personal and community group participation in the processes of the local state.

STRUCTURALISTS

The New Left entered community politics through the struggle against Rachman, the notorious landlord, in London's Notting Hill. We define the New Left as structuralist, because despite its many tendencies ranging from Marxist to anarchist, all shared in common a conception of a capitalist society where equal social relations could not be achieved without the transformation of that social order. The murder in 1958 of Kelsoe Cochrane, a young West Indian carpenter, led the infant New Left to believe that they should seek to contest the underlying issue of the housing problem and landlordism as a means of defeating racialism. As John Rex (1978) recently and autobiographically observed, (he, too, had been involved in this venture) there was perhaps a too easy belief that dealing with the material conditions which facilitated racialism was tantamount to dealing with racialism itself. None the less, this pioneering foray contained all the elements of group mobilisation, social surveys and the attempt to seek redress through legal process which were to characterise a structural (and, for that matter, many pluralist) approaches to community action.

Whilst this pioneering venture took place in the late 1950s, the next round focused not on the private landlord but on the excesses of the local state in its provision, or rather non-provision, for the homeless. The activists within the King Hill hostel struggle in Kent in 1965 came out of the militant but non-violent strand of the Campaign for Nuclear Disarmament (CND), the Committee of One Hundred. While CND was to become a vast, essentially middle-class protest movement against nuclear warfare, the support given it by the New Left in its earliest period was crucial to its survival and success.

While the struggle in Notting Hill drew in Marxists such as Stuart Hall and Raphael Samuel, and activists such as George Clark and both the O'Malleys, the King Hill struggle was activated by a more libertarian style of socialism. Andy Anderson and Jim Radford (although Radford was subsequently to be charged by the community activists with co-option for his attitude to the Piccadilly squat) were at that point the leading activists and closely associated with the group. This new wave of radical community action thus very early on had established the interest of both the Marxist and the anarchist strands of socialist theory.

Despite the debate between Marxists and anarchists as to the most appropriate theory and practice for revolution, perhaps what neither of them saw was the degree to which both were liable to be incorporated within community work as a paid activity. But so far as these contesting activists were concerned, worse was to come. As social work departments began to include community workers in their establishments in response to the Report of the Seebohm Committee, the focus of debate shifted to whether community social work is the same or different from community work, and even to whether working from one department of the local authority gives rise to 'truer' community work than work from another. While from a radical perspective these debates can be likened to that of the number of angels who can dance on a head of a pin, once community work is based on a pluralist conception of society of necessity strategic and tactical discussions occupy an intense but smaller social space.

At the same time as the debate on the nature of community work was beginning to crystallise, the government-sponsored Community Development Projects were beginning to disseminate a new analysis. Having overthrown their consensual origins (which agreed to blame the poor for the condition they found themselves in), the CDP analysis returned to a classical preoccupation of the Marxist analysis, namely the structural antagonism between labour and capital. While the point of production remained *the* place around which mobilisation was to occur, the home and neighbourhood as the loci of reproduction became of increasing salience to the discussion. Thus, the majority of the CDP reports stressed the relationship between the economy and the level and character of welfare provisions. Some of the projects began to analyse the situation of the local areas in which they found themselves in terms of the movement of capital, of the need for areas of changing land use and of transient populations. Inner-city areas are described as functional to capitalism as they enable profit to be made from changing land use and provide a source of surplus workers.

This analysis, however, neglects the fact that the primary workplace of the woman is located within the community; indeed, as we wrote in 1975, 'to study community is to study women' (Rose and Hanmer, 1975). The strategy that flows from the CDP analysis is aimed at bringing together the two sides of the paid worker's life, the home and the place of employment. The assumption is that the inroads that capitalism makes in the community and the factory can be resisted by aligning community organisations with those of paid workers, typically tenants' associations and trade unions. Women, despite the key work they perform, often remain marginal, shadow figures, behind the usually formal male leadership of community organisations. Thus in both areas of collective activity, women are seen as supporting the male vanguard, their capacity for independent action remains unrecognised, not only by the community workers but by the men and even by the women themselves.

A NEW DIMENSION IN THE STRUCTURAL CONFLICT MODEL

Despite the influence of the CDP critique which itself drew substantially on the growing political economy of the city (Castells, 1972, 1977; Harloe, 1976) the theory sat ill at ease with the personal experience of women community workers. Gradually, sustained by a movement whose epistemology affirmed personal experience as a legitimate means of knowing the world, an alternative construction of feminist theory and practice began to be forged. While it would be premature to suggest that this feminist analysis is fully developed, none the less certain elements within the critique are both increasingly identifiable and being drawn into the discussion of community work theory and practice. In order to understand these disparate elements, as the connections are far from clear, we need first to consider the experiential material generated by the women community workers, and secondly, as this is a current item on the community work agenda, to explore the contours of the debate concerning domestic labour and its implications for the labour theory of value.

Although ignored by both community work (by all three of the competing paradigms) and by the new political economy of the city, community struggle and action conducted by women became increasingly evident as part and parcel of a growing feminist movement. While the first national women's liberation conference was held in Oxford in 1970, it was not until 1975 that Marjorie Mayo, on behalf of the Association of Community Workers, began collecting articles for *Women in the Community* (Mayo, 1977), and it was 1977 and 1978 before women community workers, identifying themselves as such, began to gather. Feminist concerns were difficult to express because women community workers, particularly in, for example CDPs where the political economy critique held sway, shared the view of the domination of capital and the connectedness of industrial and community struggles. They found that both themselves and also the women they worked with were excluded from the analysis and, further, on occasion only able to work with women in their non-paid time. Somehow it was not appropriate or central enough to merit paid time being spent on work with women and in experiencing this as a contradiction, the issue of who is being oppressed by whom is raised in a new form.

To understand why work with women in the community is not 'real' community work, it is necessary to look at the analysis of the position of women within capitalist society (CDP, 1977, 1978).

Classical Marxist analysis tended to take for granted the woman's part in the reproduction of labour power; a revitalised concern has drawn attention to this and has re-emphasised the significance of women as part of the reserve army of labour. Whether the woman's work in the family realises use or surplus value (and this is under dispute in the domestic labour debate), she is not seen in her primary labour as a producer directly confronting the capitalist, as is the male industrial worker. She is, however, indirectly producing for the capitalist who benefits from her labour as she services her husband so that he can return to another day's work, and through reproduction and child care she produces tomorrow's labourer for capital. Thus the woman is said to labour for capital as does the man (albeit at one unpaid remove) and together they face a common class enemy.

Contradictions in the relationship between men and women within this tradition are seen as contradictions 'among' the people rather than 'between' the people; that is, that the antagonism which exists between husbands and wives in the context of the working-class family can be transcended through primarily ideological struggle. A type of cultural lag theory is used to explain why attitudes do not change upon a revolution in the economic base; consistent propaganda and re-education efforts may be advocated. Because there are held to be no structural problems within the working-class family that demand radical change, it can be treated as the smallest unit both of analysis and with which to work in the community. Echoing conventional stratification analysis of bourgeois sociology, women are subsumed under the family (Garnsey, 1978). Thus the analysis, while it tells us a good deal about the workings of the sexual division of labour, in a sense, glosses over its origins.

It is this predominantly Marxist view which is under attack by feminist materialists such as Christine Delphy (1978). She argues that the wife labours, not merely for the capitalist, but even more and more directly for the husband. It is he who realises the gain from her unpaid work. To Marx's question 'Cui bono?' she points an unequivocal and heretical response. Others see the discussion of domestic labour as, while important, not tackling the central issue of patriarchy. Its historical persistence in pre-capitalist, capitalist and post-revolutionary societies to date urges a more fundamental analysis into sexuality itself. Male domination rests on the control of female sexuality and reproduction, and domestic labour is one aspect of this. None the less, regardless of their theoretical orientations, women community workers have begun to think about how they work with women, what legitimates their intervention with women, and how their own personal lives reflect, or do not, efforts to change the position of women in society.

Women community workers are beginning to experience a gap between theory and practical experience. There are several major reasons for this. Feminist ideas, in one form or another, are beginning to percolate through all sections of society, but more particularly the developing materialist theory and practice begun by some CDPs has intensified conflicts within community work. On a theoretical level, materialist theory of the CDPs speaks of radical change through heightened contradictions. Community development could never do this, as it speaks merely of adjustment which serves to contain further already quiescent thoughts and feelings. And then, on a personal level, women community workers have found themselves and the women of the community with whom they worked to be secondary characters. Community development always offered a more central role for work with women. Women community workers are beginning to alternate between resentment at being consigned to work experienced as marginal and second rate, to anger at the devaluation of work with women.

The gap between theory, especially the political economy of the city theory, as developed within the CDPs and the new urban sociology, and practical understanding hinges on the denial of female personal experience. To ignore the personal is to deny the concept and experience of sexuality, of male domination, of sexism as a mode of personal and social relations, and even of economic relations within the family. The demand to accept that the culprit is out there in a set of relations that are never experienced directly is confusing for community workers who are able to relate to the felt experiences of other people's lives. Women working with women in autonomous groups – on the whole in the unpaid or semi-paid sections of community work such as Women's Aid – do not experience this contradiction as intensely as those working in a mixed setting. This is primarily because their theoretical understanding, their knowledge of 'who benefits', corresponds to the practical experience of the women they are in touch with.

The reality of field experience is that women with young children are the key 'constituency' with whom community workers actually work. An awareness of this is crucial to an adequate theory of community work. The essential contradiction, and this echoes the sense of difficulty with which we opened this chapter, is whether we are helping to generate liberating experience with women or whether we are subtly reinforcing the social relations which determine women's secondary position in society (Meekosha, 1978). An emphasis on child care, playgroups, mother and baby groups, and so on, may be reinforcing traditional roles or stigmatising women as inadequate. Alternatively, such activities may lay the basis for the identification of interests of women as women. For the practitioner as much as for the theorist, the heart of the problem lies here.

PARADOXES AND POSSIBILITIES

There is a problem for women community workers about what activities to take up as some seem more promising for the development of both a personally valid practice and theory than others. Organising as a woman around the needs of women, helping women reach an understanding of their needs, while reminiscent of community development, may have more radical potential than applying a ready-made theory that submerges the interests of women. Indeed, because of the common difficulty concerning the social class of women in both mainstream social science and socialist thought, it may be more promising to work in those areas where the theoretical closure of a 'class' analysis is of little relevance. Work around issues of male violence seems to offer this kind of practical and theoretical opportunity, as it enables misconceptions about women's social class to be overcome as *all* women are affected more or less equally by male violence whether this occurs in the home or in the street (Hanmer, 1978). As work on violence is eventually extended to include sexual assault on children, we may extend our analysis of the contemporary family as the locus of patriarchy.

In this situation, the clash between personal experience and theory makes practice uncomfortable and encourages women to move towards community development types of work. The relationship of community work to women is at best ambiguous and largely about offering services to ease the problems of the reproduction of the generations (i.e. playgroups, play schemes, etc.); it is not about challenging marital relations, which would have the effect of challenging the respective power relations of men and women in society. The nature of the contemporary family lies at the heart of the analysis of women's oppression by the women's liberation movement (de Beauvoir, 1953, Firestone, 1971). It is in the family, that particular form of social relations, where women are moulded, controlled, restricted and defeated. Thus any challenge to marriage is a more general challenge to women's subordinate role in society. Experience suggests that only those activities that help women cope through adjustment to their subordinate position in marriage qualifies as community work. The question now being posed by some women community workers is: Can feminism be injected into community work?

In this difficult context it is not surprising to learn that some women community workers are beginning to ask if they should be spending time trying to increase the understanding of male colleagues or not. Should they try to overcome or confront the derision and hostility that often emanates from efforts to expose systems where men benefit from the exploitation of women at work and at home? Or should women workers try to build a base among women creating solidarity and actions in defence of women's interests? Parallelling the debate that took place within the black and Asian communities, so that autonomous groups became a recognised aspect of the politics of race and ethnic relations, the question remains open in so far that all positions have their advocates. It is only through experimentation, new forms of practice, that the theoretical issues can become visible.

Community work's enthusiasm for practice has not been abandoned, but it has over this decade of competing paradigms been tempered by a recognition that we have to make sense of practice in theoretical terms. While this 'making sense' is enormously difficult, the gift from the feminist movement which has been so late to arrive yet so precious for structuralist community work to receive, is the recognition of the necessity to integrate personal experience with the conceptual understanding of the world.

The boundary themes discussed in this chapter arise both from theory and practice. Community development theory stresses the need for a worker to stand outside the group or community with which he or she works, while in community action personal validity flows from identification with and, even more, actually coming from the neighbourhood or interest group concerned. Thus the gift of the feminists differs substantially from that of community development which stresses personal learning and development but limits this to the client group. As we have discussed, the act of theorising itself, while focusing thought and action, may make marginal certain groups and interests and practices. Theories draw boundaries that exclude as they enclose. But set against this, practice may articulate ideas, values, desires that can reside in a part-conscious, part-subliminal way in society. Thus the act of acting creates new situations and new understandings, which theory both refines and moulds.

REFERENCES

Alinsky, S. D. (1969). *Reveille for Radicals* (New York: Random House).

Alinsky, S. D. (1972). *Rules for Radicals* (New York: Random House).

Armstrong, K. and Gill, K. (1978). The Unitary Approach: 'what relevance for community work', and 'Lessons from community work practice', *Social Work Today*, vol. 10, no. 11 (7 November).

Arnstein, S. (1969). 'A ladder of citizen participation', *Journal of American Institute of Planners*, vol. 35, no. 4.

Bailey, R. and Brake, M. (eds) (1975). *Radical Social Work* (London: Arnold).

Beauvoir, S. de (1953). *The Second Sex* (London: Cape).

Castells, M. (1972). *La Question Urbaine* (Paris: Maspero). Translated as *The Urban Question* (London: Arnold 1977).

Cockburn, C. (1977). *The Local State* (London: Pluto).
Colonial Office (1925). *Education Policy in British Tropical Africa* (London: HMSO).
Colonial Office (1935). *Mass Education in African Society* (London: HMSO).
Colonial Office (1958). *Community Development: A Handbook* (London: HMSO).
Community Development Project (1977). *Gilding the Ghetto: The State and the Poverty Experiments* (London: CDP Inter-Project Editorial Team).
Community Development Project (1978). *North Shields Women's Work* (North Tyneside CDP Final Report, V.).
Cox, D. J. and Derricourt, N. J. (1975). 'The deprofessionalisation of community work', in D. Jones and M. Mayo (eds), *Community Work: Two* (London: Routledge).
Delphy, C. (1978). *The Main Enemy* (London: Women's Research and Resources Centre).
Donnison, D. V. (1973). 'Micro-politics in the city', in D. V. Donnison and D. Eversley (eds), *London: Urban Patterns, Problems and Policies* (London: Heinemann).
Etzioni, A. (1968). *The Active Society* (London: Collier-Macmillan).
Fanon, F. (1968). *The Wretched of the Earth* (Harmondsworth: Penguin).
Firestone, S. (1971). *The Dialectic of Sex* (London: Cape).
Freire, P. (1972). *Pedagogy of the Oppressed* (Harmondsworth: Penguin).
Garnsey, E. (1978). 'Women's work and theories of class stratification', *Sociology*, vol. 12, no. 2 (May).
Goetschius, G. (1969). *Working with Community Groups Using Community Development as a Method of Social Work* (London: Routledge).
Goldstein, H. (1973). *Social Work Practice: A Unitary Approach* (Columbia, S.C.: University of South Carolina Press).
Gough, I. (1975). 'State expenditure in advanced capitalism', *New Left Review*, vol. 92 (July/August).
Gulbenkian Foundation (1968). *Community Work and Social Change – A Report on Training* (London: Longmans).
Gulbenkian Foundation (1973). *Current Issues in Community Work* (London: Routledge).
Hanmer, J. (1978). 'Violence and the social control of women', in G. Littlejohn *et al.* (eds), *Power and the State* (London: Croom Helm).
Harloe, M. (ed.) (1976). *Captive Cities* (London: Wiley).
Jones, D. and Mayo, M. (eds) (1975). *Community Work: Two* (London: Routledge).
Leaper, R. (1971). *Community Work* (London: National Council of Social Service).
Ley, C. (1978). 'Integrated Methods and Community Work' (MA dissertation, University of Warwick, unpublished).
Lonsdale, S. (1975). 'Professionalism and Community Work' (MA dissertation, London School of Economics, unpublished).
Mayo, M. (1976). 'Community development: a radical alternative?' in R. Bailey and M. Brake (eds), *Radical Social Work* (London: Arnold).
Mayo, M. (ed.) (1977). *Women in the Community* (London: Routledge).
Meekosha, H. (1978). 'No Politics, No Base, No Legitimacy – Community

Work and the Feminist Dilemma (MA dissertation, University of Bradford, unpublished).
Mitton, R. and Morrison, E. (1972). *A Community Project in Notting Dale* (London: Allen Lane).
Moorhouse, B., Wilson, M. and Chamberlain, C. (1972). 'Rent strikes – direct action and the working class', in R. Miliband and J. Saville (eds), *The Socialist Register 1972* (London: Merlin).
Nisbet, R. (1967). *The Sociological Tradition* (London: Heinemann).
Pincus, A. and Minahan, A. (1973). *Social Work Practice: Model and Method* (Itasca, Ill.: Peacock).
Power, A. (1973). *David and Goliath, Barnsbury 1973* (Holloway Neighbourhood Law Centre, Sheringham Road, London N7 8ND).
Rex, J. (1978). *Race in the Inner City* (London: Commission for Racial Equality).
Rose, H. (1976). 'Participation: the icing on the welfare cake', in K. Jones and S. Baldwin (eds), *The Yearbook of Social Policy* (London: Routledge).
Rose, H. and Hanmer, J. (1975). 'Community participation and social change', in D. Jones and M. Mayo (eds), *Community Work: Two* (London: Routledge).
Seebohm Report (1968). *Report of the Committee on Local Authority and Allied Personal Social Services* (London: HMSO).
Sinfield, A. (1969). *Which Way for Social Work?* Fabian Tract No. 393 (London: Fabian Society).
Stacey, M. (1960). *Tradition and Change: A Study of Banbury* (Oxford: OUP).
Stacey, M. *et al.* (1975). *Power, Persistence and Change: Second Study of Banbury* (London: Routledge).
Wilensky, H. (1964). 'The professionalization of everyone?' *American Journal of Science*, vol. 69 (September).
Wootton, B. (1959). *Social Science and Social Pathology* (London: Heinemann).
Young, M. and Willmott, P. (1957). *Family and Kinship in East London* (London: Routledge).
Younghusband Report (1947). *Report on the Employment and Training of Social Workers* (Dunfermline: Carnegie UK Trust).
Younghusband Report (1959). *Report on the Working Party on Social Workers in the Local Authority Health and Welfare Services* (London: HMSO).

PART TWO

CASE STUDIES OF PRACTICE

A COMMENTARY ON THE CASE STUDIES

At our request, the chapters in Parts One and Three attempt to conceptualise, to analyse, and to draw more general conclusions from past thinking and past experience. Community work practice – perhaps one should say good community work practice – is, however, highly specific and practical. The case studies are intended to provide a more human and concrete expression of the issues discussed in the chapters and a touchstone against which generalisations can be tested and improved. Generalisations are inevitably selective and segmental. The case studies will, it is hoped, provide a more rounded and integrated, even if messier, view of community work. While it was hoped that the case studies would throw light on the theme of this book, it was accepted throughout that it was more important to have an honest reporting of experience than to fit into a formula, however attractive.

What then should we look for in a case study? While this clearly depends greatly on the nature of the situation being described and the purposes of the case study, there are perhaps some broad questions which one would generally expect to be addressed. These might include:

(1) Who identified the problem and how did they define and analyse it? What factors contributed to the problem?
(2) Who determined the general course of action to be adopted? What alternatives were there? What would be the likely gains and losses of adopting any of these alternatives?
(3) What influenced the forms of organisation and communication which developed? How did people and groups come to be included or excluded and with what consequences? Was the organisation appropriate for the purposes to be achieved? How was the effectiveness of the organisation built up?
(4) What factors account for the course of the development? How did the type of population involved and the nature of the problem affect the development? What obstacles were encountered and how were they overcome? How did the broader social setting of the development affect the outcome?
(5) What were the group's relationships with other organisations? How was conflict within the group and between the group and others dealt with?
(6) What roles did the workers adopt in these developments? Were

they appropriate to the situation and the purposes to be achieved? What specific activities did the workers engage in and how did these contribute to the development, positively or negatively?

(7) What were the aims of the sponsoring organisation? How did these compare with the objectives of the workers and those of the groups involved? What did the sponsoring organisation hope to gain from the development? What did the community groups hope for?

(8) What benefits, if any, were gained from these developments? Could they have been achieved in other ways? What would have been the consequences of different approaches?

For the purposes of studying practice it is essential that the role and activity of the worker and the assumptions and thinking on which these are based should be given as much attention as the work of the target group or organisation and the development of the situation. This should include also a critical appraisal by the worker of his or her own approach and actions.

Ideally, the case study should include enough information to enable the reader to make his or her own interpretations of the situation. Such a mixture of descriptive and analytic material would also provide a basis for more general propositions or hypotheses about the practice of community work. This is a very demanding task. Potentially, however, case studies are not merely an illustration of theory developed for other purposes but an important source of an indigenous theory of practice.

In seeking the case studies for this book, we attempted to illustrate a wide range of community work activity and, despite the limitations of space, they do embrace a variety of settings, approaches, geographical locations, issues and groups with which community work is typically concerned. Inner cities, overspill estates, new towns, education, planning, personal social services, neighbourhood work, community arts, work with immigrants and the employment of local people are all represented. The weight, however, is towards community groups and local areas. Organisational change and community work at the interorganisational, planning and policy level are only touched on marginally. Mutual aid groups, women's groups, work with young people and in rural areas make no appearance, and to our regret there are no examples from Wales and Scotland. No doubt the reader will be aware of other equally serious gaps.

Participation has always been a major value of community work; more specifically community work – almost by definition – has been focused on increasing the participation of those who do not normally participate either because they do not have the capacity or resources to do so or because they are excluded. Community workers take the view that given the opportunity and appropriate support, people are willing and keen to become involved. The potential for individual and group development are emphasised and Geoff Poulton, for example, argues in Chapter 5 that: 'Control over the setting and carrying out of tasks in a neighbourhood forms a vital learning process. It should be passed on to the people involved. There is no doubt that constraints will occur as the group collectively examines its world but it will make the decision to meet, overcome or yield to forces limiting its movement.'

These constraints to participation are often denied or seen to rest primarily in the participants. Some of the difficulties are well illustrated in the case studies. In Chapter 7, Roger Else, for example, draws attention to a major obstacle when he writes that 'it is very difficult for laymen to take on professionals in situations where professional judgement is the main issue'.

Even faced by the deep divisions of Northern Ireland, the workers are able to cross sectarian lines and in Chapter 10, Lisa Huber and Felicity McCartney feel able to say that 'Community development can thus provide a bridge for the two communities to meet, as community groups in both Catholic and Protestant communities work on the same problems and issues.' They go on to point out, however, that 'a great deal of work still needs to be done at a more local and, therefore, segregated level'.

Similarly, Chris Elphick writes in Chapter 4 that 'what was needed was a new idea that involved the people of Liverpool 8 in all its aspects and that was concerned with people not problems', and he concludes: 'Obviously the community festivals did not solve the major problems facing the residents and neither did they unite the whole community, but they did bring some people together, they did help people learn new skills and develop their own creative potentials, they enabled people to develop self-confidence and they demonstrated the potential for self-help and corporate action.'

Much of the discussion of community work has in fact been concerned with the activities of workers in relation to participation and community groups. What is often denied is that in order to work effectively with community groups, workers must be effective within their own organisation and also in relation to other organisations at all levels. Lisa Huber and Felicity McCartney draw attention to the fact that: 'Major decisions and the allocating of resources which affect people most are not taken at a community level. Thus the community work strategy must work upwards as well as outwards.'

In Chapter 6 Gerald O'Hagan emphasises the importance of inter-agency work and concludes that community groups in his neighbourhood have been too busy with their own programmes at the expense of collaborative efforts and a more general problem-solving strategy.

Another theme underlying the case studies is an uneasiness about intervention. There are concerns about the legitimacy, credibility and relevance of intervention, and fears that intervention may stigmatise or create dependence or arouse false expectations or come between groups and the institutions which should serve them. Is intervention in the interests of the interveners or those that sponsor them rather than in the interests of the population ostensibly being served? As Geoff Poulton writes in Chapter 5, 'it became clear that the team were viewed with considerable suspicion. Had they arrived to carry out research, then to complete their PhDs elsewhere? Were they going to draw people into various activities and then depart after raising local expectations?'

On the other hand, too great a fastidiousness about the right to intervene and the dangers or unforeseen consequences of intervention might lead to a focus on expressed demand and the more articulate, while ignoring manifest need and the most deprived. Even within a relatively homogeneous population, there are usually subgroupings of various kinds so that the issue of who to work with remains a crucial one for the worker. The Belfast study in Chapter 10 is revealing in this respect: 'Conflict in Northern Ireland is usually seen as between Catholic and Protestant communities. However, for the community workers, the more immediate situation is the extent of conflict within the community. This would include the usual conflicts found in all areas – between various interest groups, political groupings, personality clashes and family feuds, as well as loyalties to groups which have emerged through the particular situation in Northern Ireland.'

The 'distance' between the organisation and the community worker and the population being served as perceived from either side emerges as a continuing concern in the case studies. What is the nature of this 'distance' in the realities of day-to-day work? To what extent is it inherent in the situation of intervention, particularly with deprived populations? What is its significance? Can it be reduced or mitigated or even used creatively?

One response is the appointment of 'indigenous' workers – that is people employed as community workers from the population to be worked with. The complex and contradictory factors which may be involved in such arrangements are pointed up by the Batley example in Chapter 9 by Ismail Lambat. Similarity of background clearly enabled the worker to establish relationships with the minority community and to meet a number of important needs for the community but also appears to have closed other options. The Belfast material also indicates that the appointment of indigenous workers has both advantages and disadvantages and sees a substantial support structure as an essential corollary. The employment of indigenous community workers needs to be distinguished from financial compensation for the leadership of local groups which raises different issues.

Sometimes the direct employment of the community worker by the community he or she serves is advocated as a way of reducing distance and increasing direct accountability. Some of the dilemmas which may arise in these situations are frankly discussed by Dudley Savill in Chapter 8. He concludes: 'If the staff are prepared to work on the boundary of the organisation, co-ordinating and encouraging growth, then their work can be extremely beneficial . . . However, there exists the temptation for community workers . . . consciously or otherwise to manipulate the policy of the organisation.'

This raises the question of the appropriate role of the community worker in relation to those with whom he or she is working. This is not systematically discussed in the studies or even elaborated, although the matter is touched on in a variety of ways. There seems to be considerable similarity in the activities in which the workers are engaged – investigating, collecting and disseminating information, establishing relationships, creating organisations, analysing and assessing, clarifying and developing objectives and priorities, mobilising human and material resources, planning and implementing action are evident at many points in a continuous and interacting cycle. The thinking and intellectual aspects of these activities are relatively easy to describe. More intangible but equally important is the worker's ability to establish appropriate relationships.

These are not only activities of the community worker but are also activities of the community group, and the two strands are often confused and obscured in discussion and sometimes possibly in action. How should the worker's activities relate to the study, planning and action of the group? There seems to be considerable agreement that the worker has a supportive, servicing, enabling, facilitating role in relation to the group and the individuals involved. The worker is fostering increased awareness and understanding of situations, problems, opportunities. The worker has an educational role in passing on knowledge and skills directly, but perhaps even more important by his whole manner of working and relating to people in ways which do not assume or create dependence but stimulate the capacities of the individual and groups to think and act and take responsibility for themselves.

More obscure and more problematic is the extent to which the community worker should adopt a leadership role or make decisions for those he or she is working with. There is clearly a range of practice and no doubt, given the variety of situations being addressed, different stances may well be appropriate depending on the circumstances. The situation is further confused by the fact that people appropriately in leadership positions may use community work methods. Whilst eschewing grandiose claims, Gerald O'Hagan, in Chapter 6, attempts in various ways to distinguish his role as community worker from others who contribute 'a particularly great amount of time, effort, energy, thought and imagination'. He argues that the community worker is concerned with the interrelation of specialisms and their human implications. He suggests that: 'Through having no other role and a greater available time than any one other, there are perhaps three community work processes that I perform more than any one else. These are spreading amongst others in the community and the local authority, an awareness of the community work category of problems and particularly, opportunities . . . encouraging a wide scan of the contents of the community work category of problems and opportunities; and the executing of back-up tasks.'

Although such a facilitating rather than a leadership role would seem the appropriate one for community workers, the balance in this respect will be affected by other valid considerations in the particular situation. While it may be highly educational for a group to learn from its own mistakes, this benefit must be weighed against, for example, the elimination of certain options or opportunities for the group, or even its very existence. Discussion of these issues is often complicated by the possibility that those involved may intentionally or quite unknowingly say one thing, intend another and do yet a third.

At least two of the workers explicitly define their role as a boundary one. Discussing experiences in Leigh Park, Geoff Poulton writes in Chapter 5: 'So the team were placed on the edge not only of professional workers, but also in residents' estimation. They were boundary men from the start of the Project.' Gerald O'Hagan echoes this in Chapter 6: 'My role is not any part of that central action. This is a position at the periphery of the common perception – that I share – of what the central action is.'

A further role complication arises because workers often become involved in providing personal support for some individuals and families. This is perhaps more pointedly illustrated in Chapter 9 by Ismail Lambat. Community work is concerned with collective action and activities designed to foster it. This approach is often contrasted sharply with a concern for individual needs and problems. In so far as community work is concerned with deprived and stigmatised populations, workers will inevitably be asked for personal help and the way they respond will affect their credibility. Personal needs and relationships can also affect participation and performance in community groups and this needs to be understood and coped with.

The organisational arrangements for community work are often complex and there are many permutations. Funds may derive from a number of statutory and voluntary sources, and support from one statutory source may be channelled through another, or through a voluntary organisation. Whatever the funding pattern, community work may be part of a multi-purpose organisation such as a department of local government or the primary function of an independent voluntary body. Community work may be central to the purposes and activities of the organisation or relatively peripheral. The board or committee to which the worker is responsible may be remote or close and vary from people with no commitment to or understanding of community work, to fellow workers or to representatives of the people with whom he or she is working. In day-to-day work, the community worker may be operating from a base which is distinct both from the source of funding or the employer. The people or organisations with whom he or she is working may well be yet another group. A number, although by no means all, of these possibilities are illustrated in the case studies. The question which arises is what effect, if any, these arrangements have on the role and activities of the worker and on the people and organisations with whom he or she is working.

Each case study raises issues specific to it. The commentary has attempted to bring together some themes which appear in a number of the studies. These include the opportunities and constraints of participation; the limitations of work solely at the neighbourhood level and the importance of interorganisational community work; issues of intervention; methods of relating agencies and workers more closely to the people to be served; the activities of community workers and their appropriate roles in relation to the groups and organisations they are working with and their leadership; personal problems and collective action; and the auspices, funding and organisation of community work.

These themes are neither comprehensive nor definitive, even in terms of this particular selection of case studies, let alone the field of community work generally. They are presented merely as a background to the consideration of the case studies and will have failed in their purpose if they foreclose discussion or alternative perspectives. Readers should interpret the case studies for themselves and for their own purposes.

Chapter 4

COMMUNITY ARTS AND COMMUNITY DEVELOPMENT – SOCIO-CULTURAL ANIMATION

Chris Elphick

In recent years, in many European countries, a movement has developed in the arts which is concerned with the role of the arts in our society and the relevance of cultural activities to everyday life. The Council of Europe has produced a formidable body of literature concerned with the creation of a cultural democracy – I shall deal with this notion more fully later in the chapter. A climax to this work was reached at the conference of European ministers with responsibility for cultural affairs who met in Oslo in June 1976.

At this meeting, a European Cultural Convention was signed by all present. A number of resolutions were passed and principles of cultural policy adopted. Three of these are particularly relevant to the development of community arts in this country and are worth quoting in full here:

> Cultural policy can no longer limit itself exclusively to taking measures for development, promotion and popularisation of the arts; an additional dimension of our societies reinforces respect for individual dignity, spiritual values and the rights of minority groups and their cultural expression.

> There should be an innovatory aspect in Cultural policy and encouragement for the development of a whole range of new socio-cultural activities so that all may take an active part in the cultural life of their community.

> Cultural policy at the local level should particularly aim at allowing all sections of the population to be involved in the process of change which affects them by means of a coherent policy for socio-cultural community development.

In simpler language, these resolutions refer to the development of creative activities that are not only relevant and accessible to the majority of our society but are also created by them. The last quote sets an important precedent by linking cultural activities to social change and the need for a coherent policy to facilitate that desire for change.

The term 'socio-cultural animation' is not widely used in this country, but we do use the two terms of 'community art' and 'community development'. The purpose of this chapter is to discuss their relationship, concentrating on the practice of the work rather than the theory.

It is not necessary here to attempt a detailed definition of community development, but it is perhaps important to consider briefly what may well be a less familiar term to the readers of this book – community arts.

One of the aims of community arts is to stimulate people to an active concern for the needs and aspirations of the community of which they form part. Arts-based activities, therefore, are likely to form part of community development as a whole and may very often operate within an educational or social framework. Community arts activities have something of their own to offer to the arts, something which may well change our appreciation of what art is. At their best they go beyond making more people more appreciative of, or receptive to, the established arts and go beyond a matter of taking art to the people. Community arts are fundamentally concerned with the relationship between art and people. They challenge the traditional concepts of high art and élitist culture that have tended to impose an alien minority interest on the majority of our society. They challenge the state of cultural imperialism that has existed for centuries in the UK and which has dominated and determined the direction in which cultural developments should move.

In practical terms, community arts relate to mural projects, print shops, video, film, photography, music, street theatre, crafts, creative play schemes, festivals, workshops, and so the list could go on. There is no one activity that can be described as community art – the whole range of artistic–creative activity can be included. Community arts are concerned with opening up channels of expression and communication within sections of the population where they had not previously existed; with helping people collectively to express values, feelings and opinions; with the development of personal, social and cultural awareness; with passing on skills and with the active involvement of people from a particular community in activities designed for the needs of that community.

It is worth noting here a few comments by Jean Hurstel who describes himself as a 'cultural animateur' – a man of the theatre who practises his profession not in terms of theoretical production, but in relation to a specific group of people. He goes from door to door establishing relations with inhabitants and groups seeking out the unique identity of each area. He acts as artistic adviser as they express themselves, create objects, films and plays. 'Encouraging people to meet and express themselves means putting the concept of cultural democracy into action, at least it is a modest attempt to do so' (1974). Hurstel sees the function of the *animateur* as breaking with former ossified functions and unsuitable professional structures; it introduces new practices and new methods marked by a concern for democracy, for inter-personal relationships, for popular expression. The animateur is a 'creator of exchanges, forms and contradictions'.

This statement relates not solely to community arts but to the whole field of community development. Community art, as part of socio-cultural animation, cannot be separated from community development at all. It uses different techniques but is, I believe, a creative arm of community development. It is important to recognise that other community development techniques ought to be highly creative and imaginative and creativity is not the sole prerogative of the arts.

Our society links culture to refined tastes or judgements and to high intellectual and aesthetic development and it refers to people with such tastes or who have experienced such developments as cultured. The implication for the rest of us is that we have to strive to become cultured. In order to help this process, the concept of democratisation of culture has been introduced. Here traditional cultural values are introduced to working-class audiences by the way of street theatre, plays and music in community centres and working men's clubs, and paintings on display in public libraries. The values have not changed, only the ways in which they are brought to people.

Our concern must not be with such a process but with helping to establish cultural democracy. This must be why we encourage self-expression and promote contact between groups and individuals. The establishment of a cultural democracy concerns an approach to all socio or cultural action:

> Against the social order and the reigning bureaucracy which tries to enclose all relationships within the rigid framework of rules and hierarchies, community development pits creativity and democratic decisions taken at the grass-roots; against advertising it pits consumer action and against television it sets community television and experiments in video, information and self-expression for a whole range of social groups. (Hurstel, 1974)

Cultural democracy is in total contradiction with the economic, social and cultural order. Community development expresses this contradiction. While we may be attempting to establish cultural democracy, we have not yet succeeded. It follows, therefore, that community development must be not just a methodology but a means of social change and the *animateur* a militant of social change.

Contemporary man has decided to state not his privilege but his right to be part of the decision-making which rules his life and decides his destiny. Community development is here to stay but it is essential for community developers to widen their vision. It is not only power to the people, the solving of basic social issues, the refusal to be pawns in political games which concerns a community, but also the power within a people to brighten its life, to come alive in celebration and to develop creative skills and talents. Obviously you cannot celebrate human life and experience if that life and experience is without real humanity – we must continue to fight for the cause of human dignity. But people cannot fight without arms – they need tools with which to work. The basis of all tools is self-confidence and self-respect; without these no battle can be won. Socio-cultural animation can create situations in which self-confidence and self-respect can be regained and personal skills, talents and abilities can be explored and developed. Thus community art can help to provide tools without which community development cannot take place and participation is likely to become a hollow exercise.

It was said of the community festival discussed later in this chapter that 'a community which celebrates together in harmony, may find a greater inspiration to organise itself when it comes to some of the harsher issues of living. Groups within a community which have sung and danced together may find it much easier to talk together and even argue together in a more trusting atmosphere' (Dodd and Elphick, 1974). These comments refer to the whole range of community arts activities – if they are well organised and fully enjoyed and if there is true follow-up, then they can lead to a readiness to meet the hard realities which seem so forbidding to the community.

It is impossible, in the space available, to consider in detail anything like the whole range of community art activity, but perhaps it would help readers to know the range of activities of one community arts project. The Rathbone Project in Liverpool describes itself as an experiment in education in the community, and uses a whole range of community arts activities in its work. Photography ranging from making tin boxes into pinhole cameras to mastering the art of developing and printing 35mm film; silk screen printing for posters, T shirts and Christmas cards; mural painting on gable ends, bridges and electricity substations; street festivals and carnivals; costume and mask making; puppetry including the construction of shadow puppet theatres; drama and improvisation; and environmental landscaping go towards making up this range of activities. They involve people of all ages in learning new skills, experimenting with new ideas and searchng for useful resources.

For the rest of this chapter I would like to concentrate on one event, a community festival, which not only demonstrates the variety and value of community art but which clearly shows the relationship between community art and other aspects of community development. I make no apology for using as an example events which happened five years ago. What was demonstrated then is every bit as pertinent, if not more so, today.

In the summer of 1972, Liverpool 8 witnessed what the press termed Britain's 'first race riots since Notting Hill'. Groups of young people fought each other. If the press were not using the words 'race riots', they were calling the trouble a 'housing war'. Neither of these phrases was true – violence erupted out of boredom. Young people, already suffering from unemployment, bad housing, poor educational opportunities, widespread discrimination and police harassment, were bored – there was nothing to do. The only way to use up spare energies was in violent, destructive activity at first directed towards property then towards each other. These activities were widely reported in the press and on television. Embarrassed police, social workers, councillors and corporation officials set about trying to solve the 'problem' – this being seen as the people. Small amounts of money were spent on activities to give them things to do, police held public meetings to show that they were not as bad as all that, and a community worker was employed on the estate that was at the centre of the trouble. The 'troubles' were treated as isolated incidents and not as symptoms of what was happening all around us. What else can we expect if we continue to create an unequal society, with unequal opportunity and resource distribution, that is based on privilege and profit?

By Easter 1973, many local people, especially mothers of the young people involved in the 'troubles', could see that promises made by the authorities were doing little to change the situation and that if that summer was not to see a repeat of the previous year, they had to do something about it. The question was, what? For years Liverpool 8 had been overrun by community and social workers – they had all been trying to solve the area's 'problems'. Most of the traditional methods had been tried and the people knew that for anything positive to happen, new ideas had to be tried. They also knew that traditional methods meant doing things for people usually in set categories (old, young, etc.) and that the whole area was looked at as a series of problems. What was needed was a new idea that involved the people of Liverpool 8 in all its aspects and that was concerned with people not problems.

I had been working in the Granby Street area of Liverpool 8 as a community worker since 1971 and had been closely involved with many of the young people and their parents. This involvement with the parents seemed to develop rapidly and in the Spring of 1973 I helped bring together local residents who had all expressed concern at the situation to consider what to do next. In order not to break the sequence of information relating to the festival I shall return later to consider my role as *animateur*.

We were unclear as to exactly what was needed, but we were clear that we wanted activities that related to all members of the community and that encouraged energies to be directed towards the creation of an enjoyable summer. These activities had to be freely available, imaginative and exciting – they also had to be flexible enough to allow developments to take place as the summer progressed. The summer was concentrated on because that is the time when boredom and tension seem to run highest. While we were considering what type of action we might take, BBC TV showed a film of the El community festival that had taken place in the East End of London during the summer of 1972. This seemed to us to portray the type of atmosphere we should like to see created in Liverpool 8. So the idea was born – a community festival.

Because no one really had any clear idea of what such an enterprise might entail my colleague, Pete Dodd, and myself were asked by the group to visit the people responsible for running the El festival to try to get ideas that could be developed back in Liverpool. While in London we met a community arts group called Free Form who agreed to help us. They visited the area, met and worked with the group, and July 1973 saw the start of the first community festival in Liverpool – it was also the first six-week-long community festival anywhere in the country. Many people outside the area predicted disaster – to most of Liverpool, Liverpool 8 was known only for its crime, prostitution, vandalism, drugs, etc. It often provided sensational stories for the local press. Nothing was ever written about community action, about the positive side of life in the area (it had its own community transport, housing and banking schemes), about the multi-racial character that provides so many benefits to life in the area, and so on.

Liverpool 8's first festival lasted for six weeks, cost over £2,000 and included events ranging from large-scale ones involving thousands of people, to small localised activities of a few dozen people. It covered a geographical area of about two square miles which fell into four distinct localities. The festival crossed many barriers – physical barriers (such as main roads), racial barriers, age barriers, community barriers, authoritarian barriers, etc. Again many people thought these barriers would be our downfall.

In the outset, the first Granby Festival ended after a very happy, peaceful summer in which many people of all ages, races and creeds indulged in communal fun and enjoyment.

Two visiting groups of artists took part – Temba, an African theatre group, and Free Form. These groups ran workshops involving people in a variety of creative activities. As well as teaching their skills, they gave performances in community situations (streets, public houses, community centres, open spaces) throughout the area and Free Form, in particular, staged large-scale events (Crazy Day, Fireshow). The groups also serviced street parties. These parties were a major part of the festival with every street being encouraged to run some sort of party. The festival started with a grand carnival parade and had several outdoor events including a music festival.

Festival activities were new to everyone and no one really knew what to expect. Many people in authority treated the festival with caution and the organising group[1] often had to struggle for help and support – it was a long job getting equipment, materials and finance. However, the group concerned with the actual running of the festival had great faith in each other and in what they were doing. They believed in their ideas and in the power of community activity.

The first festival ended in September, but that was certainly not the end of the community feeling it had created. In fact it was the end of the beginning. People had experienced, for the first time for many of them, a summer full of hope, enjoyment and excitement created by their own hands. Many people began to be aware of what skills they had and of what they were capable if they had the will to achieve. It was our job as community workers *(animateurs)* in the area to build upon these aspirations and to help individuals achieve what they wanted. As well as personal achievements, several communal activities were created as a direct result of people either talking to each other at festival events or being introduced to each other by members of the organising group. An important function of this group was actively to promote contact between groups and individuals (for example, residents' groups, ethnic minority organisations, etc.) where such contact did not previously exist.

8 pages, a local community newspaper, was started; Play on Wheels. a mobile play resource unit, was set up to provide play resources around the area; a couple of new residents' associations were started and Granby Resources – silk screen printing, typing, duplicating and photography facilities – was opened. As well as these material developments, it was obvious that many of those barriers mentioned earlier were crossed during the summer – the task in September 1973 was to continue to cross them in the hope that they would eventually be broken down.

It can be said that many of these activities had little, if anything, to do with the 'real' problems of bad housing, poor environmental conditions, racial prejudice and low standards of educational provision. Directly, this is certainly true but then the festival was not designed with this in mind – it achieved its aim of helping to create a peaceful but exciting and challenging summer for large parts of the population of Liverpool 8. I know that one consequence of the festival, as with many such activities, was that through coming together in an atmosphere of celebration some people remained together either as friends or as members of issue-based groups tackling some of the problems outlined above. There were many vivid examples of individuals appearing to realise, perhaps for the first time, that they were not alone in having certain problems.

The fact that there would be another festival never really seemed in doubt – indeed planning started almost as soon as the first one had finished. The organising group was still an *ad hoc* body of people from the area who had come together simply because they were interested in the idea of another festival. It contained most of the original group plus about a dozen 'new faces' who had become involved as the summer progressed. One of the first topics to be discussed concerned the type of activities that should take place. This discussion was characterised by a feeling held by most people present that they wanted to learn more and be entertained less. It was also felt that many of the ideas introduced to the area by groups such as Free Form and Temba could benefit the large number of small local organisations such as play schemes, community associations, playgroups, youth clubs, etc. This would only happen, however, if the emphasis was on skill sharing and the development of ideas, so although the second festival was still concerned with community celebration it also involved the passing on of skills and ideas relevant to other community activity that could be developed outside a festival structure.

So several more community arts groups were involved, working with music, street theatre, puppetry, inflatables, video and developing imaginative and creative ideas for the several play schemes in the area. The large-scale activities and events were modelled on those of the year before with one or two major additions. The opening celebrations spread into a weekend with the second day taking the form of a giant family picnic in the local park. Another addition was to stage an International Weekend. Liverpool 8 is fortunate in being a multi-racial and multi-cultural area. The great variety of dress, food, religions, customs and languages make it a richer place to live in – it is obvious that any festival in such an area should strongly reflect this aspect of community life. In one way this was reflected in all the events, but the International Weekend laid special emphasis on events put on by the local West Indian, Asian and African groups. Street parties were again a major feature, with more street-based activity arising from projects such as Play on Wheels and Granby Resources which had been set up following the first festival.

The organisation of the second festival showed that much had been learnt in 1973. People remembered what had happened then and were far more aware of the potential of a festival atmosphere – as a result they made the most of the situations that were created.

A festival becomes a feeling that lasts long after the actual events. People get to know each other better and an area gains a social confidence of a kind that enables its residents to deal with their environment in a more positive way. Even the local authority began to take the residents of Liverpool 8 seriously. The fact that a long, ambitious plan had been successfully put into operation by local people had demonstrated to all concerned that by working together ordinary people are a powerful force. A festival also brings out talent and ability – some people found that they had an organising ability, others found they could paint or dance, or had a special talent for helping each other. It is this revelatory, liberating aspect of community festivals, and indeed most community art work, that is the real reward and perhaps the final aim. Once people have got themselves together in a festival, the basis is laid for many things to happen. In the Granby Festival area the needs for activities with young people were examined and the potential of various ideas was explored. Because of the ideas and skills that had been developed during the festivals, the way was open to respond to needs in a more creative and imaginative way. People found that by doing things together they had more chance of success. The value found in sharing skills and ideas during a festival, the expertise that is gained in terms of action and organisation, can effect great changes in local community action.

The Granby festivals could not be labelled as only community work, community art or community education – they were examples of socio-cultural animation using a variety of techniques. Community workers and community artists were involved, along with local people, with everyone participating in a variety of learning processes. A criticism of the festivals was that they ignored the real issues that caused people to be deprived and depressed – unemployment, poor educational provision, lack of opportunity, etc – and substituted them for the icing on the cake. Some community workers felt that community arts had nothing to do with social change and that all a festival did was to divert attention, and funds, away from the real problems of the area. The festivals were labelled by some as good agents of social control. However, it was interesting, but not surprising, that all these criticisms came from people living outside the area. The local people had listened for a long time to others telling them how deprived and oppressed they were and how they should stand up and fight. What they were not told was how? It was all very well exhorting them to enter into a boxing match with the authorities, but without gloves they would be slaughtered and, perhaps of more importance, where was the team that was to do the fighting?

The people of Liverpool 8 were not together and, although often sharing common problems, rarely realised it. Obviously the community festivals did not solve the major problems facing the residents and neither did they unite the whole community, but they did bring some people together, they did help people learn new skills and develop their own creative potentials, they enabled people to develop self-confidence and they demonstrated the potential for self-help and corporate action. More non-community art activities came out of the festivals than those directly concerned with community art – in this case, community art was a starting point for the whole process of community development.

I have touched on the role played by the *animateurs* during the Granby Festival developments, but it is perhaps important to go into more detail at this point. There is no doubt that our role was essential to the development of the festival idea. We made contact with community arts groups, arranged for them to visit the area, wrote grant applications, and obviously influenced the type of activities that took place. We did, though, work closely with the other members of the organising group throughout, and had regular twice-weekly meetings at which all proposed action was discussed.

We would have been unable to work in this way if it had not been for the Neighbourhood Projects Group (a local authority-financed but independently run co-operative of community workers covering the inner city of Liverpool) who paid us and gave us the freedom to take chances and develop ideas. We all lived in the area and had done so for about a year prior to the 'troubles' that led up to the first festival. NPG made financial resources available to allow us to rent a work base and provide basic equipment.

I was particularly concerned about two things. First, I thought it would be easy for the festival itself to become the all-important thing and that the reasons why it was created would be forgotten. It was important to remember that the festival was created in response to a particular situation – once that situation changed then perhaps the response should also change. Secondly, I was particularly conscious of being in an influential position regarding festival developments and where possible attempted to discuss this position with members of the organising group.

We attempted positively to affect the situation in two ways. First, by arranging, through NPG, to employ two local residents to be actively involved with the organising of the second festival and follow-up activities, and secondly to build on the ideas already expressed that the development of more localised activities, emphasising skill sharing, was prefered to large-scale events.

The first course of action proved to be quite disastrous, owing to the fact that shortly after employing these two people, the then Liberal-controlled Liverpool City Council withdrew its grant to NPG and we were unable to continue their employment. Although remaining as voluntary workers they devoted less time to the festival than they would have done otherwise.

Ironically, the curtailment of the grant helped our second course of action. We were able to convince people that they could no longer rely on our full-time involvement in large-scale activities, but that perhaps we could all be involved in the development of more localised projects. I helped set up the Rathbone Project in part of the festival area and other *animateurs* continued to work with different projects – the community newspaper, Play on Wheels, tenants' associations, credit union, photography project, etc. Certainly in 1974 the types of activities introduced to the area through the festivals were more wide-spread although less dramatic.

I still believe this course of action was right if only to reduce the dependence by local residents on professionally involved people. It is true to say, though, that our initial close involvement with the festival idea, knowledge of the problems we were all up against and keenness to see our critics proved wrong led to us not paying enough attention to the fact that this dependence was not only possible but probable, and should therefore have been actively tackled right from the outset of the ideas. Looking back now on the situation, community art and festival-type activities still play a large part in the life of sections of the Liverpool 8 community through such channels as play, youth work, education and community development.

Before concluding this chapter I would like to add a brief word on education. I have not used that word very often here and have not referred specifically to educational activities. I consider everything that I have talked about to be educational. Education is nothing to do with a schooling process but everything to do with a life-long process of liberation, learning and achievement. Throughout our lives we all take on the role of educator. The festivals vividly illustrate the importance of sharing the roles of teacher and taught and they show what happens when this is done. Many of the activities were intensive learning processes entered into by young and old alike with energy and enthusiasm. When learning is joyful it takes on a different dimension and can only have a positive effect on our lives.

In writing this chapter, I have tried to give some idea of the value of creative activities in the process of community development. Community art is only part of the process and there will be many situations in which it will not be the relevant way of working. All community development must be concerned with vision – as *animateurs* we must have a vision of the society that our work is helping to create. Maybe that is an obvious statement, but I am continually meeting people involved in the field who appear to have no overall political or social vision which necessarily affects the work they do. My first introduction to community art was a hostile one – I took a lot of convincing that creative activities could play a part in a process that I identified with action and conflict. I was suffering from a narrow vision that prevented me from being open to suggestions of ways of working that appeared to deviate from my narrowly conceived view of community development.

I would like to end with a challenge related to training in the fields of community art and community development. When considering the work of the *animateur* we must look at what underlies this work – what animates the *animateur*. *Animateurs* encourage others to question what is and to voice desires for change. Can we do this if that desire is lacking in ourselves – have we been sufficiently challenged to relate our theories and ideals first and foremost to ourselves?

It is not enough to establish a centre for institutionalised, technical and theoretical training; a training place for cultural democracy must be created within the spirit of animation. Here, starting with the desire to question and act, people capable of tolerating contradictions, militants of social change, creative minds are educated.

NOTE

1. The organising group was never an officially constituted body but remained an *ad hoc* group of interested residents serviced largely by two *animateurs* – Pete Dodd and myself. The group fluctuated between about ten and thirty people for meetings, increasing dramatically when practical help and expertise were required. The group consisted largely of women and included several members of local ethnic minority groups – the men tended to involve themselves in practical activities rather than meetings. As well as attending meetings, individuals worked closely with us on the organising of the festival – the time they were able to give was obviously dependent on other calls on their time.

REFERENCES

P. Dodds and C. Elphick (1974). 'Community Celebration', mimeo., CETU 17–21, MVMPS, Oldham, Lancs.

J. Hurstel (1974). *Training of Animateurs* (Strasbourg. Council of Europe).

Chapter 5

A STUDY IN COMMUNITY EDUCATION

Geoff Poulton

The concept of frontiersmen moving into uncharted territory in order to study the habits of native tribes and possibly to colonise, if climate and prospects prove to be favourable, is one reserved for a rapidly decreasing proportion of the earth's surface. Yet it is a concept which hovers uneasily around the notion of community development and action research in urban and rural areas of industrialised countries. Records kept by the New Communities Project team during the first year of their work in Leigh Park, a large housing estate lying to the north-east of Portsmouth, reflect the unease felt by those involved (Fordham, Healy and Randle, 1974).

The task of the project team – two research workers and a university-based director – was to examine the provision of adult education services in an area of urban overspill and, if necessary, to seek a more effective penetration of the area by the providing bodies (the local education authority, the Workers' Educational Association and Southampton University Department of Adult Education). Attendance at adult classes organised by the LEA showed a disturbing bias towards people living in more affluent parts of Havant borough during the late 1960s and early 1970s. The bias was disturbing because, traditionally, adult education has concerned itself with provision for working-class people over a long period. A series of movements and studies commencing with University Extension in 1873, the Workers' Educational Association in 1903, through to the Russell Committee's report in 1973, pointed to the need for processes which would encourage as much participation as possible of the whole working class in adult education (Hutchinson, 1970; Jepson, 1973). The processes developed over a period of a century had not successfully produced proportional representation of students from different backgrounds, however. By the 1950s, Trenaman (1967) had shown that people classified as from 'lower occupations' were grossly under-represented in adult education classes. By carrying out a three-year, action-research programme on a large housing estate containing a high proportion of working-class families, the initiators of the New Communities Project – the director of the adult education department, the district secretary of the WEA, and officers of the LEA – hoped to gain more insight into a vexing problem for adult educators. No consultation with local residents occurred before the project was mooted. Instead, the idea came from a conference organised in 1971 by Southampton University Joint Committee for Adult Education. By January 1973, the two fieldworkers were in post with a three-year contract to carry out their exploration funded by a grant from the Department of Education and Science.

During the first six months of their exploration the project team became increasingly uneasy about their role. Initially they were faced with the task of establishing trusting relationships with people living on the estate. But to form a position of trust implies a transaction between two parties based, perhaps, on service or on a product of some kind which could be identified as usable. The problem facing the team was that their range of available products, in the form of established local education authority and university courses, was not seen as particularly usable or desirable by many local people. As they talked to residents, it became clear that the team were viewed with considerable suspicion. Had they arrived to carry out research, then to complete their PhDs. elsewhere? Were they going to draw people into various activities and then depart after raising local expectations? The residents had experienced surveys by educational institutions in the past and little seemed to have resulted.

Local professionals from various organisations, too, had limited expectations of the project's ability to influence their agencies or the people in Leigh Park. Some suggested that the residents displayed an apathy which ground down the most dynamic fieldworkers, so there was little chance that such a small team could bring about any noticeable change in the area. The estate contained nearly 40,000 people, roughly half of whom were under the age of 25. Most of the houses were owned by Portsmouth City Council, but the area lay within Havant borough boundary. Education and social services were provided by Hampshire County Council. Over the years, since the first houses were built in 1948, an insidious process of stigmatisation and inertia seemed to have overcome people on the estate. So the team were placed on the edge not only of professional workers', but also on residents' estimation. They were boundary men from the start of the project.

The primary source of unease for the team came from the project's steering committee, however. Recruited by the project's sponsors, with the exception of one member, a local councillor, all of the committee lived outside Leigh Park and were predominantly professionals from the DES, the LEA, the university, or the WEA. The combined weight of their knowledge, expertise and influence was intended to act as a resource for the team. Their expectations of the team were aligned with promotional activities for existing adult education services and with research activities which would provide quantitative data of use for future policy and planning. Meetings were held at quarterly intervals. While the committee members may not have changed very much in their perceptions of the project's task between meetings, three months can bring about considerable changes at field level, especially when work is gaining momentum. In consequence, the team became conscious of a growing distance between the committee and themselves.

The most crucial early meeting in the team's quest for acceptability was with the Labour Party Branch, at the time the most representative political organisation on the estate. The branch felt that whatever happened in the project, local interest should be paramount. The team explained that they had no intention of imposing programmes or ideas on an unwilling population, but that they wished to work with local people towards shared objectives developed jointly with them. This was accepted with some scepticism and caution by the branch, but the team had established a period of probation within which to demonstrate its commitment and interest. By September, a number of contacts with groups and individuals had been established and the team felt sufficiently confident to adopt a more public strategy. The aim of the strategy was to create a more extensive and direct process of discovering local needs. It was also intended to provide opportunities for local professionals to learn at first-hand from residents. The campaign, called 'Breakthrough – Operation Otherwise', drew upon the services of twenty-five local people, among them housewives, councillors, together with teachers, social workers and adult educators working in the area. It consisted of a week's intensive publicity carried out in the estate's shopping centres. The team and their volunteer helpers handed out leaflets, provided information and encouraged people to complete questionnaires on what they wished to see improved on the estate. Several hundred people were approached about existing and hoped-for opportunities, as well as unmet local needs. A van decorated with campaign notices was used to move street theatre actors, a pop group and helpers to meeting places during the week of action. Clubs, bingo sessions, a picket line, factory gates, public houses, were venues for meeting the public. In this way, the involvement of a much larger number of people in working with the project team became a strong possibility.

Four strands of interest were built into 'Breakthrough'. The first was concerned with publicity for existing adult classes. A thousand leaflets, giving details of courses available at different centres, were distributed in the hope of increasing enrolments. The resulting take up of places at the local adult education centre was limited to twenty-two people, suggesting that new forms of publicity may not be very crucial, in themselves. More importantly, 'Breakthrough' provided opportunities for the officials and volunteers to enter into a new form of dialogue with residents and so begin to formulate different programmes tailored more closely to local responses.

Local responses were also important in the second strand of 'Breakthrough' since it was concerned with an interest-matching service. Here the aim was to put people of similar interests and skills in touch with one another. In addition, it was hoped that the feasibility of organising non-formal learning could be demonstrated and so point to changes required by agencies to carry out the process.[1] One direct result of the interest-matching service was the establishment of a one-parent family group.

The third strand sought to test the idea that a group could form with a very tenuous predetermined curriculum in mind, yet develop in intellectually demanding and socially satisfying ways for the participants. Two discussion groups for women were established as a result of 'Breakthrough' publicity. Meeting during the day with crèche facilities for children, the groups were led by two full-time, extramural tutors on a weekly basis. Although the groups were recruited in an unorthodox way, since classes are normally advertised in brochures and students enrol at predetermined times and pay a tuition fee, they developed in a conventional adult education mode of systematically extending the knowledge and understanding of the students.

A wide range of items affecting the quality of life open to people in Leigh Park were collected to form the fourth strand of the campaign. A wishing well, built by local schoolchildren, formed the focal point for completed 'wish in' forms. Suggestions covering entertainment, sport, housing, shopping, transport, social facilities, play space and education were collected in the well. Later the team organised a public meeting to provide a forum for the views of residents to be expressed in the presence of local councillors and representatives of various agencies. Apart from the obvious educational importance of this occasion, it provided a stimulus for the later emergence of a few action groups which sought ways to improve transport, shopping and recreational facilities in the area. A further group, concerned by the poor image of the estate projected by the press, considered establishing a local community newspaper, and, with the help of the project team, successfully produced a monthly edition of *Leap* over a three-year period. These developments showed that, given sufficient encouragement and dynamic support, people were willing and keen to become involved. They tended not to be the main activists on the estate but those who were attracted by the approach and attitude of the team.

Although one of the aims of the campaign was to develop the role of the team working alongside other professionals in order to influence their operational model, the response of local people was much more dynamic and immediate. This engaged much of the team's energy and time. Nearly two years elapsed before a good working relationship was established with an interagency group of fieldworkers. In consequence, the team were drawn into co-operative action with local people and became advocates for some organisations serving the estate. By the end of the first year, the action trap had started to close, encircling the team into local commitment which became totally demanding. The result of such absorbing commitment to action with people on the estate was to distance the team from the steering committee and, to some extent, from the providing bodies of adult education, especially during the first half of the project.

It became clear that, as the team's action continued to develop on the estate, considerable changes in existing provision would be necessary before wider participation by local people occurred. The role of the team changed perceptibly during the first twelve months of the project. Initially they were observing, listening, probing, collecting data on employment, population, schools and other educational services, identifying people with whom to work, creating some space for action to occur, helping to stimulate action, immersing themselves in the politics of the estate – in sum, adopting a learning role. Following a period of concentrated learning, they became joint actors with the members of groups concerned with specific interests. With the development of action came a gradual, but growing articulation of needs by residents and the team began to reappraise the original assumption made by the project, that somehow 'effective penetration' by adult educators of a large housing estate would be achieved by promoting what was already on offer in the form of programmes and classes.

The reappraisal commenced with the assumption that adult education needed to be placed in the social context of the estate. Many of the people who came into contact with the team had very unclear knowledge of the local authority political power structures. There was uncertainty about the ownership and control of local factories, a number of which had no union membership. But pervading the whole scene in the early 1970s was the cumulative effect on residents of nearly three decades of stigmatisation by people living outside the area. This resulted in loss of personal confidence amongst residents and an unwillingness to become exposed to criticism from neighbours or from officials of the local authorities involved on the estate. The primary role of adult education here should, therefore, be concerned with helping people to gain personal power using, as a core curriculum, factors in the local environment which caused blocks in the growth of personal and collective identity. It was, of course, useless to examine and describe power structures in the area simply as an academic exercise. Awareness of personal or neighbourhood power can only come from action experience and the actions being developed in the groups established by the team were the means to this end.

So, during the second and third years of the project the team were frequently in the role of teacher/student. Learning from the experiences of local resident experts in life on the estate, they facilitated a sharing of experiences within small groups and subsequent analysis of the problems presented. In contrast with formal educational structures, where age composition, sexual variation, or levels of achievement are the result of conscious decisions by professional educators, administrators or politicians, the groups depended upon spontaneous development. Relationships between people, their feelings, attitudes, hopes and despairs are powerful forces for learning. They are the reality of life for many people and must be the starting points for any educational development including action which leads to an increase in personal or collective power.

Much of the team's daily work involved meeting individuals with a diversity of emotional, familial, employment or financial difficulties and providing a listening period which might be followed by some form of planned joint action. For many people, this period represented a 'threshold of consciousness' which had to be crossed before further and more public action could be undertaken in the company of other residents. The continuing features of the environment in which most people live are illness, depression, financial hardship, relative powerlessness and uncertainty. The educational journey for the people involved in the project commenced with these features. This starting point also represents the point at which health, social work and education services converged and it raises a question mark over the roles and attachment of fieldworkers using a similar approach. Many of the problems the team encountered arose not so much from individuals' inadequacy but more as the result of the compartmentalisation of agency functions and worker roles.

During the second and third years of the project other and more pressing questions arose for the team, however. What underpinning could be established for some of the project's growth points? What strategies of support could be brought to bear on work in the area? Support for individuals could be provided in neighbourhood groups led by key residents, who were themselves members of the original groups established by the team. In addition, a tenuous network of groups emerged on the estate (Fordham, Poulton and Randle, 1979), partly through the promotional efforts of *Leap*, partly through overlapping membership and partly because the team was involved in a number of group activities. So the concept of a group support system began to form. Help from social work students on community work placements provided the team with a route out of the 'action trap' mentioned earlier. While their commitment to groups remained high, the team had little opportunity to create enough space for their own thinking and reflection on actions in progress. Having gained a little distance, it was possible to turn attention to maintaining support after the project ended.

The team's function in trying to influence the providing bodies of adult education now became more prominent. They conducted two surveys, one to gauge attitudes of tutors in local adult education centres and the other to register the attitudes to adult education of participants and non-participants living on the estate. In addition to obtaining quantitative information, however, the team were conscious that it was necessary to involve local fieldworkers in alternative strategies which might be more relevant to people living on the estate. A network of neighbourhood groups might be serviced by a local adult education centre, for instance.

Regular meetings of fieldworkers in the area had been established by the team. At one of these meetings, they introduced the idea of street-based education groups. They established the principle that tutors could move into neighbourhoods and work with groups of people who could negotiate times, frequency of meetings and programmes of work. The team set up an initial meeting between the local adult education centre principal and a resident who was keen to try out the idea. She would recruit her neighbours to join the meeting and they would enter into negotiation with the centre principal. The team took no part in this meeting but adopted a support role for the principal, as the street-based groups became established, since he became the activist in releasing local authority resources and was pioneering a different mode of service in the area.

The street-based groups, however, were still constrained, to some extent by the limits of the providing bodies' definition of adult education. The team were conscious of the need to leave a flexible system of support at the end of the project, which was capable of developing under the direct control of local people. The feasibility of a social and educational co-operative was examined with a number of residents. The co-operative would provide local groups with supporting and linking services if required. In addition, it would encourage new initiatives by residents who wished to improve facilities, services, employment and housing conditions. It seemed important that local residents should control and run the co-operative, helped by community workers. After a year of phased negotiations in which the team played a major part in making applications for grants, and establishing a series of achievable goals with the local authority, 'Focus 230' was founded. The first sentence of the 'Statement of intent' drawn up by founder members in 1975, reads as follows:

> The purpose of the Cooperative is to encourage and enable people to move towards a vision of a caring, sharing society; to bring about the maximum involvement of groups and neighbourhoods within the area in solving the problems that concern them, in participating in the decisions that affect them and in running their own affairs.

Even in the process of establishing Focus 230, the project team were trying to build in their own obsolescence and were endeavouring to ensure that residents would hold a central controlling presence, with community worker assistance on the periphery of the co-operative. This was a far cry from the established model of adult education provision which traditionally employs a centre principal to control and run programmes assisted by part-time tutors, within a given geographical area.[2] Learning could come from the process of setting up and running the co-operative. Those involved could develop skills of establishing relationships, of listening to others, of learning to create space for individuals' and groups' personal and collective development, of translating ideas (theories) into action (practice), of communication and helping others to communicate, of assembling a knowledge base for advice, for planning and for neighbourhood development.

By committing themselves to the creation of a new agency in the area, residents would be able to demonstrate that alternative and complementary educational modes were possible on the estate. More formal courses were available at various colleges and centres in the Havant and Portsmouth areas and, having gained more confidence from activities sponsored by the co-operative, it was possible that some residents would wish to enrol for them. The fieldworkers' group who met regularly to share ideas, information and resources were also drawn into the negotiations to establish Focus 230. They saw the co-operative as a potential neighbourhood resource, rather than as a threat to their agencies' positions in the area.

During the final month of the project's original three-year period (a nine months' extension was granted by the Department of Education and Science for one research worker to collate data from surveys, etc.), it seemed important to the team that a short review of work should be prepared for local audiences. The review attempted to present key stages in the three-year period graphically, instead of using the conventional project report. It included some of the details of services for the area, showing very significant imbalances of provision in favour of Portsmouth. It also contained some of the working principles generated by the team:

(1) The growth of adult education within an area should be ecological. It commences where people are and assists their intellectual, social, psychological, cultural and political growth, using their environment as a basis for development.
(2) It is necessary to establish a belief in the abilities, a respect for the values and a reinforcement of the potential of people, whatever their class or background might be. If this principle is applied then it follows that implicit in a belief in the potential of people to achieve is the understanding that learning to control, to make decisions and to rejuvenate their own world are well within their capabilities.
(3) Control over the setting and carrying out of tasks in a neighbourhood forms a vital learning process. It should be passed to the people involved. There is no doubt that constraints will occur as the group collectively examines its world but it will make the decisions to meet, overcome or yield to forces limiting its movement. The group will establish the direction it wishes to take; however a delicate balance is necessary between guiding the early stages of a group's life and providing longer-term physical or intellectual support.
(4) A flexible support system should be available for groups to use as required. There are resources in many areas such as rooms for meetings, materials for creative work and communicating, people with expert knowledge in specific subjects. There is often some difficulty in making them available for *ad hoc* groups, but a flexible, officially recognised support service is possible, especially if the groups themselves provide advocates to seek such support.
(5) Neighbourhood organisations should play an active part in conveying their particular message to audiences of their choice through media most fitted for the occasion. It is extremely important that people in local organisations are encouraged to present their ideas to others, irrespective of the outsider's status. The process can help to enhance the consciousness of individuals, and underpins the inherent confidence which the professional worker has in the group concerned.

The roles adopted by the team changed considerably during the project. In contrast to most action-research programmes the team was responsible both for research and action elements in the work. Initially there was a period of intense learning about the area which led to some ambivalence about the direction to be taken by the team – whether into further and more sophisticated research of educational provision or towards action. After a relatively long period of action commitment with people on the estate, during which time there was increasing reflection on the action by all concerned, the team began to be more objective and developed theory related to the work. From a base of action and related theory, the residents and the team were able to negotiate for further action, equipped with some quantitative evidence on the provision of services to the estate. During most of the project the team were providing personal support for some individuals and families as well as for some groups to a degree which is not usual within the formal adult education system. In a small way, however, they were able to show that with some initial help, people are capable of consolidating their own networks for learning, most of them outside the boundaries of the formal educational system. The challenge for the formal system is whether it can allow its representatives to cross its boundaries and run the risk of losing them to a more dynamic but irrational prospect in community education.

NOTES

1 The term 'non-formal' is now part of adult education jargon describing programmes which are set up in response to particular neighbourhood needs on the terms of the participants, in contrast to 'formal' education which has structured requirements of entry, progression, timing, fees, etc.
2 The most notable exception is the national literacy campaign 'Right to Read' which uses a process of matching tutors to individual students, often in a home-based service.

REFERENCES

Fordham, P., Healy, L. and Randle, L. (1974). 'Involving the non-participators in adult education', OECD occasional paper (Paris: OECD).

Fordham, P., Poulton, G. and Randle, L. (1979). *Learning Networks in Adult Education* (London: Routledge).

Hutchinson, E. M. (1970). 'Adequacy of provision in adult education', *Adult Education*, vol. 42, no. 6 (London: National Institute of Adult Education).

Jepson, N. A. (1973). *The Beginnings of English University Adult Education* (London: Joseph).

Trenaman, J. M. (1967). *Communication and Comprehension* (London: Longmans).

Chapter 6

PLANNING THE OPENING OF A NEW ESTATE

Gerald O'Hagan

In 1967 Camden Council completed its purchase of the site for the Alexandra Road Estate. In 1968 the plans for the redevelopment were finalised. In 1972 the last of the residents were moved out and the old houses knocked down. The redevelopment will be completed in 1979. When completed there will be 520 units of Camden Council-owned accommodation. These will house approximately 1,680 people at a density of 210 people per acre. The development also has 106 new flats not owned by the council. The local authority-owned units are built as one seven-storey and two four-storey terraces. These three terraces are parallel to one another. Between the two four-storey terraces will be a four-acre grass space. In addition, the development includes garages, shops, workshops, a play centre, a youth club, a community centre-style tenants' hall, a school for handicapped children, a social services reception and assessment centre, a social services home for physically handicapped adults, and a public works depot.

The development is being completed and brought into use in phases. At the time of writing, the play centre, the four-acre grass space, the workshops and 348 units of local authority-owned accommodation are yet to be finished.

The Ainsworth Estate is immediately adjacent to the new development. Ainsworth consists of 180 flats and is thirty years old. It is owned by Camden Council. The overall architectural strategy of the Alexandra development seeks to include Ainsworth as part of the new environment.

Alexandra Road is in South Hampstead. Two-thirds of South Hampstead is council estates.

PROBLEMS AND OPPORTUNITIES

The redevelopment of Alexandra Road presents a number of categories of problems and opportunities. A 'category' of problems and opportunities is a particular cluster of related problems and opportunities. Some obvious categories with relation to Alexandra Road include physical planning matters, architectural matters and estate-management matters. I suggest there is also a category that in a sense has no subject matter that is exclusively its own. Rather, it is about the other categories. Its subject matter is the human implications of the sum of and the interrelation between the other individual categories. I refer to this category as the community work category. This is not to say that the other categories (for instance, architecture) do not take into account the human implications of their own specialiisms; rather, I argue it is helpful and useful to 'pull out' all the human implications into a separate category.

I readily agree that this community work category is what others may variously prefer to call the sociological, social, political, human or Christian perspective. But I argue that so far as Alexandra Road is concerned, the designation, 'community work category of problems and opportunities' is at least as helpful and useful as any of these other designations.

Both the way the 'community work category of problems and opportunities' is about the other categories of problems and opportunities, and also the fact that there is a variety of alternative names for referring to the same things as the community work category, may perhaps contribute to the elusiveness of what community work is about.

The community work category of problems with respect to Alexandra Road are:

(1) The impact the new development has on the surrounding community and particularly Ainsworth. This impact is exacerbated by the already high density of population in South Hampstead and the disruption and dislocation the area has already sustained through other recent redevelopment. In addition, South Hampstead is short of play space and general youth provision, and while the provision of these on the new development is significant, it will probably not even meet the capacity and need of the newcomers.
(2) The very existence of the newcomers could be annoying living proof to established local residents of the problems in (1); there is a possibility of the newcomers feeling unwelcome. Also, simply the close proximity in which the newcomers live to each other could create stress.
(3) Problems over boundaries and territory could arise between different interests and buildings on the development.
(4) There is complexity in having a number of council departments with responsibilities for and a stake in Alexandra Road but no

special brief to work together over the human side of the problems.

The community work category of opportunities with respect to Alexandra Road is an opportunity to deliberately counter those general human problem areas outlined above as the community work category of problems. Whatever methods and processes are entailed in this countering can count as community work methods and procedures.

A necessary step in countering these problems was to engage some of those people involved within the problems. In this case, that meant contact with long-established local people and the newcomers, and also with local government officers in all the council departments with a stake in the development. I shall say more about what this amounted to after a consideration of role.

COMMUNITY WORK ROLE

Since September 1975, I have been employed by Camden Social Services Department as a community worker in South and West Hampstead; as such, community work concerning Alexandra Road has been one of my high priorities.

To be in a community work role with respect to Alexandra Road is to be aware of the community work category of problems and opportunities and deliberately to seek to act to counter the problems. It is possible to be in the community work role without necessarily having as wide a scan of the contents of the problems and opportunities as I have described in the previous section. I am the only person with the title 'community worker' involved in Alexandra Road. But I am not the only person who assumes a community work role there. However, I am the only person involved who has no other role there.

Three other people give a particular great amount of time, effort, energy, thought and imagination to being in an Alexandra Road community work role. These are the chairman of the Ainsworth Tenants' Association, a priest who lives in the neighbourhood and who was parish priest of All Souls Church until early 1978, and the curate of All Souls Church. All Souls Church is right next to the east end of the development. Unlike me, these three people have also different and important roles that embrace Alexandra Road and its surrounding neighbourhood. The tenants' association chairman's roles include latterly being mayor. And as chairman of Ainsworth Tenants' Association he is also the leader of an important interest group, although it is not by virtue of his being leader of an interest group that I am saying he assumes a community work role. Both priests are active as priests. While I am involved in other community work projects in South and West Hampstead, it is always in a community work role.

Other local authority officers and members of the local community sometimes step into a community work role over Alexandra Road.

What, then, distinguishes the 'professional community workers' from these others who adopt a community work role? Well, I have no role other than community work and I am paid to spend a full-time working week being a community worker. Both of these facts open up the way for me having more time than any other to try to put in effort, energy, thought and imagination to community work on Alexandra Road.

Through having no other role and a greater available time than any one other, there are perhaps three community work processes that I perform more than any one else. These are spreading amongst others in the community and the local authority an awareness of the community work category of problems and, particularly, opportunities with respect to Alexandra Road; encouraging a wide scan of the contents of the community work category of problems and opportunities; and the executing of back-up tasks. I shall have more to say about back-up tasks later.

The common perception in South Hampstead of what the action is all about in the Alexandra Road redevelopment is: the creation by the council of long concrete terraces of housing and some other buildings, where that leaves those living nearby, and where that leaves the newcomers. All the following have central roles: the new residents, the other residents of South Hampstead, the architects, the housing department estate managers, and the staff in the specialist agencies on the development. As professional community worker, I am neither personally affected by the development nor responsible for either its creation or the management of any part of it. My role is not any part of that central action. This is a position at the periphery of the common perception – that I share – of what the central action is.

CHRONICLE OF EVENTS

The theme of my part in events was set by my predecessor, Simon Lowles. In early 1975 he contacted housing department officers and active members of local community groups and asked them for their views on the new development; he suggested that local people and the housing department should make an effort to welcome the newcomers and devise solutions to the incipient problems.

One outcome of this initiative was that he helped the parish priest of All Souls Church to call all those contacted to a meeting about Alexandra Road. This meeting took place in June 1975.

In September 1975 my predecessor left and I took up the post and went off on visits to his contacts in order to try to get the feel and size of the pitch. One fact that had come to light through the June meeting was that the Ainsworth Tenants' Association had been discussing the implications of the development for some time. So, the chairman of the Ainsworth Tenants' Association and the parish priest jointly called another meeting in November 1975. About thirty local people and the head of the housing department's estate management division attended. The meeting was on a cold Friday evening in All Souls church hall. The intended agenda for the meeting was to discuss practical ways of welcoming and problem-solving that had been aired earlier that year and specifically at the June meeting. At the November meeting, one particular point that was discussed was the feasibility of 'building in a community of tenants' to the new development; the idea being that at the time the estate first opened, some tenants in South Hampstead on the housing department transfer list could be moved on to Alexandra Road and that this would build in some cohesion and stability.

But the bulk of the November meeting was taken up by negative reaction to the development. This negative reaction had three parts. First, the points I have set out under (1) in the list of problems in the section on problems and opportunities. Secondly, some fantasy beliefs that grew from anxiety about the real problems; such a fantasy was a belief that the reception and assessment centre was really a borstal. Thirdly, was the objection that such a development was under way at all; these objectors would have preferred the old Alexandra Road to have been rehabilitated or replaced by a similar road of town-houses.

Literally, a cry came from someone in the meeting: 'Why don't we have an exhibition about the new Alexandra Road?' This sounded like some sort of opportunity to grapple with the first two parts of the negative reaction. So, I undertook to follow up the suggestion. On that slight note of optimism, the meeting ended.

The Alexandra Estate Exhibition took place in South Hampstead on four evenings in June 1976. The exhibition consisted of a model of what the new Alexandra Road would look like and plans, sketches and descriptions of the different types of buildings. The exhibition was staffed by senior officers from the architect's department, the housing department, the social services department (the director himself on one evening), the chief executive's department, and the Inner London Education Authority. These officers were kept busy answering questions about various aspects of the estate. About 400 local people visited the exhibition. The majority of the people I spoke to on those evenings saw the new development as an unwelcome change. However, all were pleased that at least the exhibition let them get an idea of how South Hampstead was being altered. The minimum the exhibition achieved was to show the surrounding community that at least the council cared enough to make an effort to show properly what it was doing; this aspect, of course, was an exercise in communication rather than participation.

Ironically, the planning and communications department declined to be involved in the exhibition. But all the other council departments with some responsibility for the development contributed time and effort to the exhibition. These efforts were co-ordinated and produced into the exhibition by the public relations division of the chief executive's department.

There was an unplanned and, I think, extremely important spin-off from organising the exhibition. An *ad hoc* committee had met a few times before the exhibition in order to work out exactly what we were doing. Regular attenders were the parish priest and the tenants' association chairman (as conveners of the November meeting which had called for the exhibition), myself, the public relations representative, and the senior responsible officers from the architect's department, the housing department, and the ILEA youth service (for the youth club). I suggest that what happened was that council officers in this group – both by being with those other council officers who had different departmental briefs towards the site and by being with three people (the tenants' association chairman, the parish priest and myself) who had an Alexandra interest but not a specific brief – saw the development now no longer just in their departmental terms but rather in 'whole' terms. They reflected on the challenge the development posed to local people and the newcomers. Put another way, they appreciated the community work category of problems and opportunities.

At the last meeting of this *ad hoc* committee before the exhibition, the head of the housing department's estate management division suggested that the group continued to meet after the exhibition.

Taking up this suggestion, the tenants' association chairman and the priest convened the first Alexandra Estate Committee in October 1976. That meeting appointed the priest as chairman of the committee and adopted the following terms of reference:

(1) To help the new tenants feel welcome and settled down.
(2) To encourage a sense of neighbourliness.
(3) To identify and ease any possible areas of conflict.
(4) To consider the effects of the estate on surrounding neighbourhoods.

(5) To provide an information service between concerned and responsible parties about what different departments and people are doing on the estate.

The Alexandra Estate Committee is an expanded version of the exhibition organising committee. At that October 1976 meeting, the headmistress of the special school, a senior officer of the reception and assessment centre, a senior officer responsible for the play centre, the warden of the pensioners' flats, the social work patch team leader, the estate manager designated for Alexandra, and the new curate joined the committee. The housing association pensioners' flats were just opening. The school and the reception and assessment centre were not ready to open until 1978, but it was possible to contact the headmistress and a senior reception and assessment centre worker because both establishments were transferring from other sites. The committee meets for a couple of hours on Thursday afternoons about every six weeks. The number attending varies; a dozen is an average attendance. Additions and changes in membership occur. The committee has decreed it will disband around the time when the last newcomers arrive.

The overall function of the committee – both outside and inside the meetings – is sharing of information and ideas and co-operation over tasks in order to try to create a pleasing new human environment. After the committee ceases to meet, I believe the regular attenders will continue to perceive themselves as and interact as members of a network; the sum of this network is the local government responsibility for this new slice of South Hampstead.

Specific accomplishments of the committee include:

(1) The implementation of a policy of housing transfer, whereby preference was given to about twenty-five families who were already council tenants in the vicinity of Alexandra Road and who were on the transfer list when the first 172 housing department-owned homes were begun to be occupied in January 1978; these twenty-five were transferred to Alexandra Road. Members of about half a dozen of these families took up prominent roles among the first new Alexandra Road tenants as welcomers to and communicators about South Hampstead.
(2) The preparation, in autumn 1977, of a leaflet which consists of a map of the new development and a list and description of all the new buildings on Alexandra Road. This leaflet was distributed to homes around the estate and was available at the nearby Abbey Community Centre and All Souls Church. The leaflet is also given to all new Alexandra residents.

(3) The preparation, in January 1978, of a 'Neighbourhood Guide for Alexandra Estate Residents'. The guide has information about local schools, play and children's leisure provision, public transport, shopping, advice and consumer services, entertainment and recreation, libraries, doctors, dentists, health clinics and places of worship. The guide also has a map of the estate in relation to its nearest main roads. Every new resident receives a copy of this guide.

(4) In September 1977, a wide range of people involved in any sort of helping role in South Hampstead were invited to a special evening open meeting of the committee. About fifty guests attended; these included the Ainsworth caretaker, the beat policeman and a doctor. The aims of the committee were shared with those present.

(5) The committee pressed London Transport for an increase in local bus services during the rush hour to allow for the newcomers. A slight increase was provided.

(6) In February 1978, the committee held a 'meet the neighbours' evening at the new tenants hall. This was in honour of the occupation of most of the first 172 units of Camden housing department accommodation in January and February 1978. All the residents of Ainsworth and all the newcomers to Alexandra Road (including the non-council flats) were invited. Three hundred people came. They met each other and talked to members of the committee. About twenty-five of the people came from Ainsworth; they mostly still saw the new development as an unwelcome disruption. All the newcomers I spoke to were delighted with their new homes and environment.

(7) The member of the committee from the reception and assessment centre staff explained to the committee just what her agency is. The warden of the pensioners' block of flats then asked this residential social worker to repeat the talk to a meeting of the pensioners. The pensioners' block is next door to the reception and assessment centre. This talk to the pensioners took place. At it, some fears were allayed and plans laid for children from the centre to visit some pensioners in their flats.

There are other community work initiatives about Alexandra Road which did not originate in the committee but were brought to it for the information of others. For instance, the tenants' association chairman and the architect organised tours of the building site for interested local people. Also, the tenants' association chairman works to develop the new tenants' hall as a genuine hub of the local community.

BACK-UP TASKS

The chronicle of events is the shape the community work opportunities have actually taken. Some of the tasks involved – for instance, attendance at committee meetings – are obvious ones. But a number of tasks not obvious from the chronicle of events were nevertheless necessary to establish the legitimacy of and to innovate and maintain the momentum of the initiative involved. I refer to these as back-up tasks. I believe I perform more back-up tasks than any one else. This leaves me with a significant responsibility for establishing the legitimacy of and innovating and maintaining community work initiatives.

Negotiating is a key part of these back-up tasks. Significant negotiations include:

(1) Suggesting and arranging that the tenants' association chairman and the parish priest jointly convene the November 1975 meeting; this was the start of a fruitful partnership.
(2) Encouraging the estate management officer to attend that November meeting; this helped create fuller involvement of the housing department.
(3) Persuading the different local government departments to commit resources and time to organising the exhibition – and especially persuading the public relations divisions to do the nuts and bolts of co-ordinating the different contributions.
(4) Discussing with the different members of the exhibition organising committee what the estate management officer's suggestion to continue meeting could mean and who else could be usefully included.

Other sorts of back-up tasks include:

(1) Drafting letters of invitation to the November 1975 meeting and writing and displaying posters for it.
(2) In partnership with the parish priest, writing the terms of reference of the Alexandra Estate Committee.
(3) Acting as secretary to the Alexandra Estate Committee by taking and distributing the minutes, drafting and sending letters, and writing and distributing the 'Neighbourhood Guide'.
(4) Producing and helping distribute leaflets for the inaugural tenants' association meeting of the newcomers.
(5) Arranging for and participating with newcomers in the making by silk-screening of posters to advertise events in the new tenants hall.

Back-up tasks support and underpin the main effort of the community work strategy. They act on the main effort. To that extent they are on the periphery of this main effort. When they fall to me to perform, they contribute in an extra way to the peripheral position of my professional existence.

EMPHASIS

In 1975, I thought my main emphasis over Alexandra Road would be neighbourhood work. However, my main emphasis has in fact been an interagency one. One reason why this has happened is simply that I have learnt more about the possibilities of interagency work. But another reason is that I am an active neighbourhood worker in South Hampstead and as such my opinion is that community groups there have been in general too busy with their own programmes and/or (like the local public at large) too antipathetic to the redevelopment to want to be part of a problem-solving strategy.

I may increase my neighbourhood work input to Alexandra Road as more newcomers arrive.

My relationship with the other agencies (such as the architect's department and the housing department) is characterised by a marginality. I am not a member of their professions or departments. I share none of their central responsibilities. Yet by the way I help present some of the factors, we have together occupied a common ground of opportunities.

EMPLOYER

I enjoy being employed within a social services department. I work from a social work area office and share a room with two colleague community workers. My employer pays for its community workers to have a consultancy service. I feel integrated within the fieldwork effort of the department.

However, the department's senior management did veto an otherwise successful piece of negotiating by the social work patch team leader and myself with the housing department for the temporary use of a flat on the Alexandra Estate, to act as a neighbourhood patch base for social workers to be on hand as the newcomers moved in.

But I gauge that colleague social workers do consider wider social work ways of working, simply by being acquainted with community work initiatives in their patch. This, combined with a serious intention by social workers to develop a patch system of working, has meant that I feel my work over Alexandra Road has some positive influence at a field level in the department.

Chapter 7

COMMUNITY WORK IN A NEW TOWN

Roger Else

I joined Milton Keynes Development Corporation as a community development officer in July 1970, soon after the publication of the master plan for the new city. This plan proposed the development of houses, factories and facilities for 250,000 people over a thirty-year time scale, in north Buckinghamshire.

Development corporations, unlike local government authorities, have no direct political representatives. They are responsible to the Secretary of State for the Environment. He appoints the members of the boards of development corporations, approves planning proposals under the New Towns Act and authorises expenditure for roads, houses, factories, etc.

Decisions about most policy issues in Milton Keynes are made by the executive management committee of chief officers. Major policy-decisions are ratified by the board.

In 1970, building had been started and about 200 people formed the core of the development corporation. They comprised architects, planners and engineers; most of them organised in four inter-disciplinary teams designing different areas of the city and also central departments concerned with finance, engineering, architecture and social development, part of which was community development.

Initial Priorities

Because we had been appointed so early, it was possible for the community development officers to become involved in much more than the traditional new town activities, of helping newcomers to settle in. We were able to draw up a list of activities and allocate priorities, which would change over the years. These were roughly as follows:

(1) Work with old-established residents.
   (a) Explaining the planning proposals which affected them and helping them to query and change proposals which they considered inappropriate.

   (b) Forming self-help community services: and building up a pool of people who were experienced, for example, in running playgroups, and who could pass on their skills to newcomers in time.
(2) Working with planning and architectural teams within the development corporation.
   (a) Advising on structure plans and housing layouts.
   (b) Planning community facilities, such as meeting places and playgrounds.
   (c) Feeding back and interpreting information from residents about plans.
(3) Working with new residents, after the first houses had been built.
   (a) Visiting residents on arrival to give the relevant information about their locality.
   (b) Helping to form groups and associations.
   (c) Monitoring the difficulties which residents encountered and helping them to sort them out.

The activities show a bias towards planning, with 'participation in the planning process', a high priority. This approach met with approval in the development corporation (it was shortly after the publication of the Skeffington Report) and most people genuinely felt that public involvement could make a positive contribution to the planning process. It was after all, a goal of the master plan. For two years, all community work took place in the existing settlements.

As a community development officer, most of my time was spent outside the main office, working with residents. Inside, I divided my time between, on the one hand, working on various social policy issues, with the in-house social development staff, and, on the other hand, working with planners and architects in the area design teams.

With both camps I was able to develop strong social and professional relationships. Having discovered their jargon and the ways in which they operated, I felt competent to put over my own ideas and to interpret to the professionals the ideas and aspirations of residents.

The social development unit, like most other sections, never carried an overridingly strong voice in development corporation decision-making, but it did give many opportunities for innovation and for constructive criticism of development corporation policy.

During my four years in community development, I became involved in a wide variety of issues, most often at my own initiative and usually working alone, though with the support of the community work team which I lead, which consisted eventually of twelve full- and part-time workers, and of senior officers in the social development unit.

In this short account, it will be impossible to describe everything which went on and I have selected two topics, one concerned with physical planning in the established townships and the other with city-wide roads and transport policy.

THE LOCAL PLANS FOR NEW BRADWELL AND WOLVERTON

Early in 1971, the development corporation published a booklet containing outline structure plans, with tantalisingly little detail, for all the established towns.

Some of the most significant proposals related to New Bradwell, a small town of about 2,500 people, built originally towards the end of the nineteenth century. Whole streets of the town had been scheduled, without consulting the residents, as redevelopment areas. Hardly anyone read the booklet and many of those who did so did not realise that redevelopment meant that their houses would be knocked down and replaced.

The document had been prepared and written before I joined the development corporation and the social development department had not been consulted. When I discovered the proposals, I consulted my contacts in New Bradwell, chiefly two local councillors and arranged, with them, a number of meetings with residents in the scheduled areas. There I explained in detail what the booklet proposed and what the effect of those proposals would be upon the residents. The elderly were particularly horrified by the main proposals and two groups immediately sprang up to raise petitions to the development corporation to save the houses.

I helped the groups, using my typewriter, to compose letters for them to take around for signatures. At the same time, I worked within the development corporation to question the plans with the people who had made them. It was clear that no one had looked closely at the houses, but had assumed from a cursory glance that they were substandard.

When the petitions reached the development corporation, signed by everyone, I briefed the social development officer and the general manager. I also prepared a report describing the situation in New Bradwell and putting forward arguments for preserving most of the houses. The arguments, supported by the petitions, were accepted in principle and the chairman, general manager and local board members visited residents to see for themselves the state of the houses, which were, on the whole, in excellent condition.

Soon afterwards, the development corporation made a statement that the streets would not be redeveloped. It was an easy victory and I decided to take advantage of the euphoria, by suggesting that the residents should now decide how they wished New Bradwell to be planned.

We arranged two further meetings in the village hall, at which thirty to forty residents at a time sat in groups of six or eight with large-scale maps of the town and felt pens. A number of issues arose, concerning the lack of car parking, children's play, sheltered housing for the elderly, canal safety, general recreational facilities, allotments, etc. I encouraged residents in their groups, to replan the town as they saw fit and then to discuss their proposals with other groups, making trade-offs as necessary, until a consensus appeared.

After the meetings, I fed all the information back to the planner and architects at the development corporation, who had just started to look at the town. They welcomed the comments and many of them were incorporated into the plan, which included a General Improvement Area.

It was during this process that some local councillors began to complain that the council itself had not been consulted and that my activities were in some way undemocratic. My superiors in the development corporation, however, argued that they valued this direct consultation with the residents and that the council would be consulted formally in due course. The councillors accepted this, allowing me to continue, though I was asked to keep a 'low profile'.

With the planners and architects, I helped to arrange a large exhibition in the local workingmen's club, which more than 1,500 people attended. They were pleased with the plan and enjoyed meeting the architects and planners. I spent a lot of time helping residents to understand the proposals, and incidentally making more contacts in the town. A great many extra comments and suggestions were made and these again were incorporated, where appropriate. A good deal of the improvement work had now been completed and residents are at present negotiating with the development corporation, the borough and the county council, to turn the obsolete junior school into a community centre and workshop.

A similar procedure was contemplated for Wolverton, but the larger size of the town (7,000 people) and a rather less cohesive community made it less successful. Local councillors were also more active and the whole process was much more formal. The effect of my involvement was minimal, except in commenting on the proposals and advising on the presentation of material for the exhibition.

Public participation in the planning process is usually an extremely difficult exercise for planning officers to do effectively. The most successful attempt which I made, in New Bradwell, treated participation as a means of teaching residents about planning; presenting the issues and helping residents to understand the implications of them; leaving them to decide amongst themselves about priorities. Patience is all important and I found it most useful not to be too involved in the planning process myself; to act rather as a teacher, and messenger.

Some professionals can cope with direct contact with members of the public. One of our architects was introduced to a group of housewives interested in the functional aspects of house design. Together they designed a housing estate which has proved to be very popular with residents. I helped the group, with two of my colleagues, to gain sufficient confidence in their command of the necessary skills over many months, before they began working with the architect. It was, however, an isolated example and has not been repeated recently.

Working in a development corporation removes some of the pressures found in many local authorities. Because he or she is not responsible directly to a committee of members, a community worker is often much freer to approach residents without treading on the toes of their local councillor. In New Bradwell, where councillors had safe seats and welcomed participation, there was no real conflict. In Wolverton, where the political atmosphere was more intense and where councillors were rather more suspicious of the intentions of the development corporation, it was much more difficult to get significant numbers of people involved. Councillors felt that their traditional role was being usurped and they put pressure on the development corporation to keep community workers at arm's length.

THE TRANSPORT USERS' GROUP

Not long after new residents began moving in, it became apparent that public transport services, which had been reasonably adequate for the established townships, could not cope with the needs of people who were living on the more isolated estates. One of the community workers in my team gathered a group of residents on one of the estates. I invited them to my community office to discuss their problems. Most of them were housewives with small children, who found it difficult to get to the district shops and services. Together with another resident, who was a lecturer at the Open University with access to video equipment, we made a short video-tape illustrating the problem; this we showed, with the housewives, to the planners, architects and engineers responsible for the area.

The film made its point to those who saw it, but they had no direct means of influencing the transport authority. I then contacted a number of other residents, whom I knew to be interested in transport planning, and arranged further meetings with them and the housewives to plan a campaign to improve services. There appeared to be two different approaches. One was the direct negotiation of revised services with the bus company. The second, and more radical, was an appraisal of the basic master plan for the city, to discover whether it could ever permit an effective public transport system, or whether the plan should be altered to accommodate public transport more efficiently.

Calling ourselves the Transport Users' Group, we began by looking at the first option and the group invited the area manager of the bus company to meet them. We discussed with him the difficulties that members of the group had encountered. He in turn presented the difficulties which he found in providing services. The session ended with the bus company agreeing to relocate some stops and to put on a new pilot service to an outlying hospital. The transport users agreed to mount a publicity campaign, pushing bus timetables through letter boxes on their estates and publishing articles and details of transport services in their local community newspapers. My part in the activity was that of facilitator and encourager: arranging meetings, making available rooms, etc. All the initiatives in contacting the bus company came from the group.

I again met the housewives separately. They appeared to be reasonably satisfied by the response which they received from the manager of the bus company, but decided that they did not wish to take any further part in the activities of the group which was now considerably reduced in size. It was developing into a pressure group, with little popular support. As we had found with the housewives in the group, few people understood the concepts of the master plan, or were interested in them, though some of us met members of residents' associations in an attempt to enlist more support.

We continued meeting in various members' houses to plan the campaign. Most group members, who were university lecturers and other professionals, knew at least as much as I about the subject and my role was less of a leader, rather someone with a thorough working knowledge of the plan who could keep the group informed about current corporation policy and changes that were imminent.

To prepare my own position, I talked to development corporation staff concerned with planning roads and transportation. I found, in general, that the planners and road engineers were totally committed to the master plan and to preserving the integrity of the planned road network. The public transport section were, however, more sceptical. They were not completely convinced that a satisfactory public transport system could be operated.

I considered, therefore, that my intervention into what would clearly turn into a fundamental criticism of corporation policy was justifiable and necessary – from the point of view both of the users' group and of the development corporation itself.

At first, the group examined in detail the many documents that had been produced by the consultants who had prepared the master plan. A great deal of technical evidence was collected to illustrate various flaws which the group had identified in the plan for roads and public transport. I assisted by supplying information, most of it available to the public from the development corporation library. To begin the campaign, members of the group individually wrote letters to the local papers, explaining why they felt that the proposed city plan was incompatible with a good public transport system.

There is no standard mechanism at the development corporation for consultation with members of the public. The group had no wish merely to join in a public relations exercise with the information officer and I advised that they should write to the general manager, spelling out the arguments which had been developed. This they did.

The pre-publicity through the local newspapers paid off and the general manager wrote back inviting members of the group to meet him and other chief officers for discussion of the issues. Before the meeting, we all met to prepare our case. I advised everyone of the divergence of views at the technical level and of the approach which I considered would be the most effective with the general manager.

I attended the meeting but my position was ambiguous. The chief officers were not aware of my direct relationship with the group, but assumed that I was there because I was the community development officer with a specific interest in public participation. This suited me, since it meant that no one in the development corporation would be likely to put pressure on me to leave the group should their arguments become too vociferous for comfort.

I contributed relatively little, leaving the discussion to the other group members but interjecting occasional questions to clarify or confirm points which arose. The meeting opened up a general dialogue, questioning the apparent contradictions which we had discovered in the master plan. The tone of the meeting was generally calm and constructive. Both sides appeared to concede that the other had something to offer, but one or two members of the group appeared frustrated by the bland professional statements of some chief officers.

After the meeting the group members were on the whole pleased with the progress made, and I encouraged them to keep up the pressure of the campaign ready for a second meeting which we had arranged. Because our numbers were small, we wanted somehow to attract wider support. Yet the very limited time available to any of us made it impossible to contact all the community groups in the city.

We decided to prepare a booklet in an attempt to make our views on the very complicated issues available to a wider audience. Everyone involved in the initial research contributed a short article. I was asked to use my modest artistic abilities to draw illustrations throughout and to provide satirical cartoons. I arranged for a graphic artist in the development corporation information unit to lay out and typeset the material. I also persuaded the deputy head of the local secondary school to prepare offset litho plates and to print the booklet. We hoped to have it ready and distributed before the next meeting with the development corporation. It was, however, late. On the morning of the second meeting, the group arranged a press release of the booklet. We also presented copies to the officers at the meeting. This time the discussion grew much more heated. The officers felt that they were being pressured by the group, particularly since immediately after the meeting they were to face local journalists at their own regular press conference.

Again no one was concerned at my presence. The group fixed on what they saw as a major flaw in the master plan: its inflexibility and its inability to cope with much lower private car ownership rates. The user's group were calling, essentially, for a complete redesign of much of the city then undeveloped.

Neither side had a wholly convincing argument and after two hours of sparring, the meeting broke up. The chief planning officer was called upon to make a review inside the development corporation of the flexibility of the master plan, to examine how various public/private transport options could be accommodated.

This time, the group felt that they had achieved much less and that the development corporation officers were in such a strong position that they need concede little. As part of my wider job, I had been making contact with other workers in the field of planning and community work. In this way, I came in contact with a small firm of young planning consultants who were then working for community groups elsewhere in the country. In an attempt to use them to strengthen the group's hand, I brought them to meet the users' group. We gave the consultants all our material and asked them to draw up and cost a brief for a fuller campaign. Everyone was very keen to go ahead, but we were unable to find the finance necessary for the work they suggested. We decided instead to wait for the report.

The planning department report was predictably reassuring for the development corporation, calling for no major redesign of the master plan. Though it did make a number of recommendations along the lines of those the users' group had advocated; removing some of the planned roads and reducing the standards of others.

By this time, the campaign was running out of steam. Neither the press publicity nor the booklet had really generated any public support for the group and the members were now much less enthusiastic. Some of them had, in any case, started, with my support, on a new practical project – a Community Transport Association.

At this point, most of the users' group gave up the campaign. One or two of the members switched to a movement to question the need for an urban relief road, to almost motorway standard, of the A5 through the middle of the city.

The Community Transport Association was welcomed with open arms by the authorities. The association collects secondhand furniture and transports it at a minimal cost to the many poorly off families who have moved in with no furniture of their own and very limited means of buying anything new. It has received a great deal of help from the development corporation and now has an annual turnover of around £25,000, runs two large vehicles and employs seven people, paid by the job creation scheme of the Manpower Services Commission.

CONCLUSIONS

It is very difficult for laymen to take on professionals in situations where professional judgement is the main issue. The Windscale inquiry and the many fights over motorways appear to bear this out. Public participation is most likely to achieve its goals where issues are reasonably clear cut; where residents are directly affected and motivated to take action themselves; where positive alternative approaches can be made to planners; and where practical schemes can result.

Even more necessary, the cynic might add, is the condition that the authority being challenged should be able to make concessions which do not cause it to lose face. The development corporation had nothing to lose over New Bradwell and gained a great deal of goodwill from the residents by promising not to redevelop. Any concessions to the Transport Users' Group would have caused the development corporation to question the validity of a master plan to which it was (and is) wholly committed. Since the user group had little public support, the corporation stood to make little political gain by changing the master plan significantly. The issues were not sufficiently clear-cut and the users' group's proposals insufficiently positive or practical to be immediately acceptable to the development corporation.

It was, therefore, not surprising that the development corporation took little note of them. The group was, however, taken sufficiently seriously by the corporation to warrant special meetings with chief officers and for limited concessions to be made following the planning department reports. On the other hand, the response of the corporation to the practical Community Transport Association project was enthusiastic and immediately helpful.

Chapter 8

COMMUNITY GROUPS AS EMPLOYERS
A STUDY OF THE ALHE

Dudley Savill

'Participation' – this word attracts more nonsensical writing than any other word in the English language, except 'ecology'. However, if there is one person who cries out for participation in a perfectly genuine sense, it is the 'tenant'. Thus stated Anthony Crosland in 1973. The Association of London Housing Estates (ALHE) is an organisation which provides tenants with a forum for participation. It is one of the few large-scale community work agencies controlled by member groups employing a large staff. The organisation has a budget of over £100,000 obtained mainly from local authority and government grants. Furthermore, the ALHE musters an enormous amount of voluntary help from its members to support the various needs of some 200,000 council and housing association tenants.

HISTORY AND DEVELOPMENT OF THE ALHE

The organisation was first formed under another name by thirty-five groups in 1957. It was renamed the ALHE in 1965. The groups felt that forming a federation would help to solve their mutual problems. At the time tenants' associations faced severe difficulties with a lack of venues to meet, no help from housing departments, plus considerable hostility from the authorities. They turned to the community centres department of the London Council of Social Services who agreed to act as a helping agency with a member of its staff, Ilys Booker, seconded to serve as organising secretary.

The ALHE concentrated on providing advice, guidance and support in building up the strength of member groups. There was a long period of stability in the 1960s as the organisation established itself and became recognised by authorities, particularly the Greater London Council. However, caution was the keyword when it came to participating in political campaigns such as the East End rent struggle with the Greater London Council in 1968. But by the early 1970s when the Heath Conservative government introduced the Housing Finance Bill, which would fundamentally alter council rent levels, the ALHE was less tentative. It acted quickly in leading the protest movement against the Bill and became nationally famous in the process, emerging as by far the most articulate voice for the nation's council tenants.

As a result of their effectiveness in this pressure group role the ALHE doubled its membership from 100 to 200 estates in three years. But such growth had its dangers. The organisation showed signs of becoming a bureaucracy out of touch with the estates. Radical changes were needed. So moves were made towards decentralisation and 'borough groups' were formed. There are now ten such groups covering eight borough council areas, the Greater London Council estates and the Peabody Federation of housing association tenants. However, these groups became so immersed in tackling 'local issues' that they neglected to be involved in the ALHE's central policy-making body, the executive committee. This resulted in many of the groups' representatives excusing themselves from attending the executive committee meetings. Therefore, the reporting back of what activities were occurring in the boroughs by the groups was poor to non-existent.

The groups which are federations in their own right tended to ignore directives from the ALHE and went their own way in negotiating 'tenancy agreements' and 'consultation machinery' with their borough councils. This weakened the ALHE's scope for campaigning on central matters because it could not count on the wholehearted support of the borough groups. This caused a crisis of identity within the organisation. The issue was whether the ALHE's policy should be determined by a small 'representative' democracy or by a 'participatory' democracy. This has been partly resolved by the implementation of further 'structural changes' (ALHE, 1977). These enable the borough groups to have a decisive role in the running of the organisation and in influencing of future policy directions. The success or otherwise of this move will depend upon the relationship and effectiveness of the borough group to the affiliated estates.

LEADERSHIP OF THE ALHE

The ALHE has a tradition of working through the collective leadership of its members. It has five honorary officers who are involved in the day-to-day management of the organisation. They would be the point of contact for any urgent decision which might arise between meetings. This position has enabled the ALHE largely to develop without being dominated by the 'charismatic' leaders who are so often involved in personality clashes resulting in a fragmentation of a movement's aims. Nevertheless, this form of collective leadership can sometimes be ineffective and thus become very dependent upon the support of staff. At such times, the leadership can be very open to influence and can provide community workers with considerable scope for determining the goals of the organisation. Therefore, a staff with a common political and ideological stance could manipulate the direction of the ALHE and thus endanger its credibility. This can only emphasise the need for the democratic structure of the organisation to be strong in checking the accountability of staff.

Only recently the organisation did, for a period of eighteen months, have a chairman with a strong personality whose individual style of leadership made him very much a catalyst. One of the things he did was to challenge the role of community workers within the organisation, their influence on policy and their accountability to the executive committee. He insisted on producing his own policy documentation outlining proposals rather than relying on staff to do it for the committees. However, the moment he stepped down from the chair the ALHE returned to a collective leadership.

ROLE OF TENANTS IN THE ALHE

Tenants can become involved in the work of the organisation through various channels – by direct election on to the executive committee at the annual general meeting; by nomination to the committee through their borough groups; by participating in inter-estate activities.

One of the ALHE's biggest problems is the level of 'tenant' involvement in its work since they have a considerable workload to undertake from the estate level upwards. Julia Craddock has measured the activity level of tenants in their voluntary work. She states:

> It must be remembered that tenants' representatives carry out their work in the day and attend committees in limited spare time . . . Some tenants' representatives were found to be members of so many committees that their spare time appeared overcommitted . . . 42% of the 49 tenants interviewed estimated that they often spent more than twenty hours per week on tenant affairs. 39% were members of 5–10 committees. (1974)

The dedicated members of the organisation make a vital voluntary contribution to the work of the ALHE. They also have the exacting role of management over a large staff team. They must select workers, agree terms and conditions of service, evaluate staff performance and deal with disciplinary procedures. Until recently a specific sub-committee was responsible for management matters, referring recommendations to the executive committee. This arrangement proved reasonably satisfactory until disputes over salary differentials started escalating. This was not surprising since tenants were expected to make judgements on pay scales which were often higher than their own as employees elsewhere.

ROLE OF STAFF IN THE ALHE

The staff can be divided into three categories:

(1) There are the administrative workers dealing with the daily management and budgeting of the organisation, as well as supplying information to members.
(2) The fieldworkers functioning as enablers, brokers and advocates, co-ordinating the activities of member estates within and outside of borough federal groups.
(3) The specialists operating across the whole spectrum of the ALHE, in particular fields such as 'work with the elderly' and 'youth and recreation activities'.

The staff have weekly meetings which vary from discussions on policy matters affecting the organisation to reporting on the work they are doing. Once a month an additional session is held to study in depth case material or specific issues. These tend to be long and exhausting: twelve meetings spread over four months were spent debating proposals for the restructuring of the organisation.

The tenants differ in their attitudes to and have varying perceptions of the staff's community work role. Since the community workers are employed as secretaries of the central committees and federal groups, most tenants expect them to implement decisions arising from meetings. This includes drawing up, signing letters and resolutions, the contents of which could conflict with the workers' principles and advice. Racialism and 'problem families' are two such sensitive issues. Should the community worker decline to sign the letter or resolution on behalf of the group, he or she could be subject to disciplinary proceedings.

This functional role of the worker tends to undermine the enabling role he or she has with the group. For example, if a group is deciding to pass a resolution calling for the 'concentration of problem families', the worker intervenes by trying to get the tenants to consider the implications of 'scapegoating', it is possible that he or she would politely be told to carry out the committee's instructions as its servant! : 'You don't have to live with the problem as we do.' On the other hand, if the worker has a well-established relationship with the group he or she may be allowed to develop their theme. After all, this should be the role of the community worker. This example illustrates that within such a structured position (worker employed as an officer of the group) there is confusion in the minds of both tenants and staff of the community worker's role.

WHO INFLUENCES THE ALHE'S GOALS?

This issue has been one of the most heated areas of debate within the ALHE. I would assess that most of the 'activist' tenants involved in the ALHE believe that they determine policy decisions while acknowledging the assistance received from the staff in reaching them. Moreover, they would claim that the 'democratic structure' and collective leadership of the organisation must necessarily limit the influence of the staff.

However, there are a small number of tenant activists who are concerned at the influence of the staff. This was clear in the recorded transcript of the oral evidence of the ALHE's delegates to the Wolfenden Committee (1976), in which the following was noted:

> There is some anxiety that the staff come to be what could be called an 'Inner Cabinet'. This causes some elected members to be concerned that the staff have too much influence on policy but this is a healthy tension in any active organisation and ultimately staff are responsible to elected members.

Later on in the same transcript the tenants acknowledge that 'the flow of information is controlled by the staff and there are times when the staff need to act quickly and independently'. (ALHE and Wolfenden Committee.)

The main protagonist of the view that the staff controlled 'policy making' was a tenant, Mr. X, with more than ten years' involvement in the work of the ALHE. He raised this issue a number of times over the span of two years at various committee meetings but never found any real support. However, he was incensed by an article appearing in the ALHE newspaper *London Tenant* (1976) written by a senior member of staff under the title 'Participation and all that'. This article raised a number of questions about 'consultation' and 'participation' schemes and was written from a critical point of view: 'Participation in general is fraught with difficulties. A majority on a committee with little power is in many ways worse than useless because it can create an impression of power without reality and as such can be dangerous.' Mr X, having represented the ALHE as one of two members on the housing management committee of the Greater London Council for three years read this as an attack on his involvement in 'participation'. He wrote a letter to the editor of *London Tenant* (1976) but because of the serious nature of the contents the executive committee vetoed publication. The concluding paragraph of his letter raised a number of queries.

> Is the Association of London Housing Estates getting value for money? Are the staff as efficient as they could be? If not, then the staff have a duty to put their own house in order, after all, there is little point at casting stones at tenants' representatives until they are absolutely sure that they themselves are blameless. The Executive Committee are responsible to the membership for forming policy. Should staff members make policy matters for which they are not responsible and for which they cannot be called to account? This is a matter of interest and concern to us all.

Mr X who had been for three years an officer of the ALHE and for many years a member of the executive committee resigned from the organisation. He did so mainly on his belief that the staff were influencing decisions through an inner cabinet politically motivated. However, he was to some extent a lone voice in the wilderness but he raised a number of valid questions. His mistake was to credit the staff with being a 'cohesive' team and for misjudging them as a 'political cabal'.

The issue he raised of who runs the organisation is very much a pertinent question. Certainly the staff, then a much smaller group, played a key role in the ALHE's campaign against the Housing Finance Act. There was a very strong identity by the workers with the tenants in fighting legislation so deeply rooted with 'social injustice'. It was not a time to stand back and be non-directive. There was no place for the workers to operate on the periphery of the tenants' movement, they were either out of it or totally committed to the battle. John Hayes assesses the part played by the staff in the campaign:

> The General Secretary as head of the staff team was in great demand as a speaker being respected as a dedicated worker for the tenants' cause. Many estates appreciated his advice, encouragement and leadership. He had the responsibility of conducting the campaign and co-ordinating the efforts of both staff and tenants. (1978)

At the time Mr X was discussing the issue of 'staff influence' there had been a considerable turnover and a notable increase in the number of workers. The staff was by no means a 'homogeneous' group. The new team contained several individuals whose ideologies, philosophies and experience varied widely. They were not a group to be easily welded into a cohesive team. This unstable position clearly undermined their influence during the long-drawn-out debate on the restructuring of the organisation. This was a crucial exercise of consultation between tenant members and staff on the future direction of the ALHE. The staff, far from initiating possible avenues of change, found themselves on the defensive, unable to reach a consensus on agreed objectives. There is no doubt that a united team with the experience, knowledge and background of the ALHE staff could not only exert a strong influence but could determine the shape of the organisation's goals.

ISSUES OF CONFLICT

There was one issue of conflict between the ALHE as an employer and the staff which dominated my period as general secretary. This was the question of line management and the role of general secretary as the 'hierarchal head' of the staff. Soon after my arrival at the ALHE in 1971, I had discussions with the staff team, then consisting of seven people, to work out ways of reducing pay differentials. It was also clear that as I had fourteen different areas of responsibility, some delegation was crucial. It seemed to me that the most effective way to rectify both problems was to enable the staff team to operate as a co-operative. My objective was to build an organisational structure allowing all the staff to achieve the greatest possible job satisfaction with equal financial rewards.

I received the support of the staff for the proposal but encountered total opposition from the tenants of the executive committee. They argued that it had always been the tradition of the organisation to have a 'hierarchal' chain of command which to them had always functioned well. It was necessary for someone to supervise the running of the office and the fieldwork. Since they worked at their own jobs during the day they had limited opportunity for monitoring the management of the organisation. They, therefore, needed to be confident that someone was co-ordinating the activities of staff members. It was easier for them to relate to an individual rather than a number of people. The tenants saw no need for change in spite of constant staff representations.

Realising that I should not influence the tenants to accept the co-operative principle, I set about introducing a 'collective system' of staff decision-making. Each individual had an equal right to express an opinion on an issue and each had equal power in the reaching of decisions. I divested myself within the staff team of a leadership role and shared out a number of responsibilities, such as supervision of fieldwork. It was agreed that the administrative unit would deal with the appointment of secretarial staff. We worked out methods of narrowing pay differentials. I agreed to put the case to the appropriate committee.

This particular item caused the tenants much consternation. There was some irony. It meant that I, on the top salary scale, was arguing a reduction in level of increments to myself, whilst pressing for an increased level for workers at the other end of the pyramid. The acceptance of this produced the desired levelling up of salaries which were reinforced when the committee agreed for staff to be put on local government pay scales providing that the increases could be obtained from our funding organisations.

In 1973 I left the organisation to continue my studies for a year. On my return I operated the 'collective system', but the tenants made it clear that they still held me responsible for overall management of the office and for any malfunctioning of the system. They accepted, albeit reluctantly, the collective principle in regard to team matters, but became increasingly unhappy as developments began to go wrong. Their continued questioning contributed to loss of staff morale. Furthermore, there were a number of other factors which did not contribute to the success of a collective system within the staff. I would define these as

(1) the growing size of the staff team;
(2) the uncertainty of the organisation's future due to cut-backs in public expenditure;
(3) a lack of co-ordination and direction from myself;
(4) structural difficulties allowing no clear basis for staff decision-making to be sorted out.

One of the staff team members wrote a paper assessing the problems and asserting that there had been no real evaluation on the best method for creating an effective organisation structure for a 'collective system'. The result of this was that

> on the surface issues are discussed openly together but what in fact happens is that those with personalities that can dominate, like to dictate the terms on which other members may contribute. The effect is that those with forceful personalities struggle between themselves to have their own particular terms accepted; the others become frustrated observers.

A series of incidents undermined staff confidence further. This led them to reach agreement on the role that my successor as general secretary should assume. The first paragraph of the job description stated: 'The General Secretary will be required to provide overall leadership and co-ordinate the activities of the staff team. He/she will convene a monthly staff meeting which is a forum for collective decision-making.'

The tenants of the executive committee were quite specific about the role of my successor. At an executive committee meeting (1977) held soon after my departure, members assessed the damage caused by a lack of leadership of the staff team. The recurring theme of the discussion was that 'there had been a fundamental management weakness, there should be someone within the ALHE who acts as a "boss", who makes decisions'. There was one dissenting voice who argued that the terms 'boss' and 'hierarchy' were the wrong words to use and that a new system of 'staff' involvement in the organisation needed to be considered. But the tenants had made their views clear, reaffirming a 'hierarchical' system of responsibility within the staff and reinforcing the leadership role of the general secretary.

CONCLUSION

The ALHE has evolved into one of the country's largest organisations employing community workers. Far from being affected by economic constraints, it has embarked on a sizeable programme of expansion bringing more staff under its wing. The developing relationship of the tenants and staff will have an important bearing on the direction and growth of the organisation. The relationship has been fraught with difficulties, some of which I have outlined in this chapter, but it has worked and produced impressive results.

The ALHE is twenty-one years old and is at the stage of moving from a 'representative' to a participatory democratic organisation. This process will only be achieved when the ALHE gains a much wider constituency base on the estates thus attracting a far greater contribution to its work from the membership. It is at a vulnerable period of development where much experimentation could easily fail. The ALHE is therefore even more dependent on the support of an experienced staff capable of pulling together as a team.

If the staff are prepared to work on the boundary of the organisation, co-ordinating and encouraging growth, then their work can be extremely beneficial. They have already contributed much to the organisation's high standing and credibility in local government circles. However, there exists the temptation for community workers to become too closely identified and involved in the tenants' movement. Such a strategy can lead staff consciously or otherwise to manipulate the policy of the organisation. This could be counter-productive, with the effect of damaging the tenants' interests. There must be a strong monitoring system which can effectively check any abuses, but at the same time encourage the mutual growth points of community workers and tenants working in harmony.

REFERENCES

ALHE (1977). *An Introduction to the ALHE.* A booklet on the organisation obtainable from ALHE, 17 Victoria Park Square, London E2.

ALHE and Wolfenden Committee (1976). Recorded transcript of meeting between representatives of ALHE and the Wolfenden Committee on Voluntary Organisations held on Tuesday, 24 February 1976.

Craddock, Julia (1974). *Tenants' Participation in Housing Management, A Study of Four Schemes* (London: ALHE).

Crosland, Anthony. Speech to the Standing Committee of Parliament dealing with the Housing Finance Bill.

Hayes, John (1978). *The ALHE and the Fair Rents Issue* (London: ALHE).

The London Tenant, no 3 (July 1976).

Minutes of ALHE executive committee meeting held on Saturday, 3 September 1977.

Chapter 9

COMMUNITY WORK WITH AN ASIAN COMMUNITY

Ismail A. Lambat

I propose to discuss the community work I was engaged in among the Indian Muslims of Batley in West Yorkshire. My aim is to convey the experience of the work, rather than to present a complete analysis.

The work was undertaken over a period of two years. The first few months of the work was done as a member of the Batley Community Development Project and the rest as a member of Batley East Ward Project, which consisted of three workers employed by the local authority, Kirklees Metropolitan Council, in the immigrant area of Batley.

Batley is a small town with a population of just over 40,000. In the past it was very closely associated with the shoddy and mungo trades and, to a lesser extent, with textiles. By the time the Indian Muslims came to settle, both the town's industries and physical condition were in various stages of decline. Despite this, and attracted mainly by the abundance of cheap housing and a quiet atmosphere, the Indian Muslims chose to live there and work in the neighbouring towns. From the early 1960s their numbers grew and now stand at over 5,000 persons. They live almost exclusively in a few streets of the town, in the East Ward. This area consists of the oldest, mainly back-to-back housing in Batley, and the East Ward is one of the most deprived wards in the Kirklees area.

From its inception in 1972, Batley CDP started taking an interest in the Indian Muslim community and developed some contacts with its members. It also employed a Sikh woman student for a short period of time to gather information on the local Muslims. One of the research workers had carried out a short sample survey of Indian Muslim households; in order to gain background information, its first director had visited a number of Indian villages from where the Muslims in Batley had come. Besides these activities, the project had rendered advice and information to a few individuals and had some sections of the welfare benefits literature translated into Gujarati to make it accessible to those who could neither read, write nor understand English.

After I joined the project the language and socio-cultural difficulties that existed between it and the Indian Muslims were eased because I was from the same ethnic group as most of the local population. Most of them came from landowning families in India, who traditionally were at the top of village hierarchies. There were also Mullahs (hereditary priests), barbers, village messengers and weavers. The traditional occupations continue to play a very important role even when the occupation itself is no longer practised. They are also a sensitive issue in a situation where people are trying to rise in the social scale. For example, a person belonging to a traditional group of barbers will keep to his group, by entering into a marriage within his group, but he will not like to be called a barber. This means that when advising on jobs, or even in casual conversation, the community worker has to be careful

In contrast to the Sikh woman appointed by CDP, I had the advantages of being a Muslim man appointed to work in a male-dominated Muslim community. And my own religion and background were similar to those of local people. I attended the mosque regularly. I also lived in a terraced home in the most run-down area of Batley and in the heart of the Asian settlement. Most important of all, I spoke the same language as Muslim Indians – Gujarati. I was also fluent in English and Urdu.

I had known some of the local people in India or had known some of their relatives. In other cases I had seen the villages or towns they had come from. In a few instances I had known or met the relatives of those who lived here, either in South or East Africa.

I did not feel that my education entirely separated me from the members of my community. There was no doubt that the people knew I had education, but my practical experiences helped me to remain close to the lives of local people. After leaving school I had started, like most other Indians in South Africa, as a shopkeeper. I took my matriculation examination as an external candidate. However, I was not allowed by the Minister for Internal Affairs to enter university. I returned to my native village in India and became a farmer. I enrolled as an external student for a BA degree and after obtaining that degree I became for two years, a full-time student for an MA degree in sociology. After this I joined a Dutch sociological research team in Gujerat and subsequently studied in Holland. Thus my studies were interwoven with several years of practical experience. It meant that in Batley I could play various roles and discuss a range of issues with the people with whom I worked. I consider this to have been of some importance.

Despite these factors in my favour, and the contacts that existed already between the project and the Indian Muslims, I had no expectations that the Muslim community would automatically accept me as a community worker.

Fears for my acceptance came about essentially for three reasons. First, four men from the local Indian Muslim community had applied unsuccessfully for my post. Two of them were from a Gujerati village which was well represented numerically in Batley. Furthermore, both the applicants were closely related to one of the most influential and respected of the local leaders. He came from a large family and also had eight married children in Batley, all with big families. If this man felt offended by not getting one of his relatives into a white-collar job he could, if he wished, tell many people to stay away from the project and myself.

The second reason for my having doubts about being accepted was that I was being brought in from 'outside' to a job which was highly regarded by local people because it was in Batley. The number of Muslims in Batley who became white-collar workers remained small because most people did not want to leave Batley. Those who had applied for the CDP job, and their relatives, had a reason to feel bitter about an 'outsider's' appointment in this sense, not because I was an outsider to the culture or religion of the community.

Finally, there was the possibility that I would be seen to be someone who would bring about significant changes in the local community. This was, of course, an accurate assessment, but those with vested interests had particular reason to be anxious. The few men with education and standing served a variety of the local community's needs. Two of them performed functions such as filling in forms and accompanying people to solicitors, for a fee. The others charged no fees for their services. They had a standing in the community and by helping those who needed assistance, they strengthened their position in the community. These men also might encourage people to be hesitant in offering their support to the project and myself.

CONTACT MAKING

These fears about acceptance started receding once I had started introducing myself to the local leaders as well as all those I could meet. In the first two weeks after taking up my appointment, I went out in the evenings and at weekends accompanied by two friends from my village who lived locally. They usually briefed me on the persons I was to see, and so helped me in preparing for the different persons I met. I also met many others at the mosque where the men gathered for their prayers. Weddings and other occasions, such as when someone was going on, or returning from, a visit to India or on a pilgrimage to Mecca, also provided me with excellent opportunities to meet people. Illness, bereavement and funerals were the other occasions when more contacts could be made and old ones strengthened. Once I got to know who the local leaders were, I kept visiting them regularly, both to develop and maintain contacts as well as to know more of the local Indian Muslims and the problems they faced.

Though I knew a lot about the Indian Muslims in general, I had to learn about the composition of the Indian Muslim community in Batley. This was essential for my work because I felt that I should know something of the persons I spoke with. Some of the information that I sought may not sound very important to other community workers. I must emphasis again that, since I belonged to the same broad ethnic group, I had to have information, among other things, on the traditional occupation group a person belonged to. Not knowing this particular item of information could lead to embarrassment both for the community worker and for the person he was trying to help. I also found out, in broad terms, the educational backgrounds of the members of the community. Attention had to be paid not only to their secular education attainments, but also to their religious knowledge.

I also sought information on the organisations to which the Indian Muslims belonged. I found that there was one organisation, the Muslim Welfare Association, to which all the Indian Muslims belonged. This association was actively involved in looking after the religious needs of its members. Despite its limited function, it was an important power base. Over the years, some of the members had become spokesmen for the community on various issues. There were other organisations, but they were village-based as membership was limited to people who came from the same villages. The only other bodies to which the Indian Muslims belonged were the trade unions at their places of work.

I soon came to learn about the problems the Indian Muslims faced. Some of the problems were particular to the Batley area, especially poor wages and poor working conditions in the textile mills. Other problems were of a general nature, such as poor housing. The Muslims faced problems peculiar to them too: what was served for school dinners, what dress girls should wear for their physical education lessons, and how and when their dead should be buried. Other problems were faced by them as immigrants registering under the Nationality Act, obtaining British passports, and arranging for their dependants to join them. As well as these problems, they had language difficulties. A sizeable number had major difficulties in communicating in English.

The initial intention was to work through existing groups, and to try and help organise new groups. However, I gradually came to work more with individuals than with groups. The reasons for taking this approach were as follows:

I could never say 'no' to the callers who started approaching me. Refusing to help an individual would have done enormous damage to my relationship with the Muslim community, as well as harm the reputation of the project because news of the refusal would have spread in the community. I was also not in a position to decline to deal with some types of work that the callers wanted done. As a community worker, who was perceived by local people as an educated person, I was supposed to know everything. Hence, whatever problem was brought along had to be looked at. Most of the problems that the callers had could only be dealt with on an individual level. I could also not refuse help to the callers because I was the only Asian community worker in Batley.

We shall see later that the formation of groups, where they were thought to be feasible, did not succeed. Working through the existing organisation was also difficult. Hence, instead of trying to say 'no' to the individuals or trying to organise groups around specific issues, I decided to make the best use of the situation by helping the individual callers and by spending time with them in explaining the problems they and others faced. I felt this to be an appropriate exercise because most of the callers lacked the 'know-how' of the causes of their problems and also of how to get them solved. In following this approach, which I would describe as a form of social education, I knew that whatever I said or did for the individual would reach many others. This permeation effect was expected because the Indian Muslim community is a very close one. Whatever problems an individual had were usually discussed between relatives, friends and people from the same village. Help and discussions with individuals were bound to filter through to various groups of persons.

The problems with which the individual callers sought help were many. The assistance requested by individuals entailed giving information, filling in forms, writing letters to official bodies and phoning for appointments. It meant explaining something on behalf of the caller, accompanying him or her to employers to sort out problems at work, to the Department of Employment, Department of Health and Social Security and DHSS tribunals, solicitors, and courts.

A record of the callers was kept for the second year of my work. The following table shows the callers and the reasons for their calling:

	Issues faced	*Callers*	*Total number of times called*
1	Employment	104	196
2	Trade union	16	43
3	Housing	185	518

4	Immigration	200	590
5	Education	64	96
6	DHSS	176	534
7	Social services	5	8
8	Inland revenue	143	230
9	Marriage counselling	6	19
10	Interpreting	23	41
11	Miscellaneous	124	240

Two things stand out from this recording: the dominance of problems associated with immigration, housing and DHSS claims, and the high rate of return by the callers on most issues. It indicated to me in particular the anxiety among many immigrants about the content and procedures of immigration legislation, and their need to turn to an accessible source of advice and information.

WORKING WITH GROUPS

I encountered difficulties when trying to organise groups from two sides. Among the Muslim people there was reluctance to involve themselves. They were too busy, were indifferent, or did not want to play a leading role. Even when some of them showed interest in discussing the various problems, when the time came for action most of them backed out. Furthermore, most of them would not commit themselves without their organisation, the Muslim Welfare Association, being involved. Yet this body was mainly instrumental in seeing to the religious needs of the people and was basically not interested in other activities. Secondly, the office bearers of this organisation were hard-pressed for time and could not undertake additional or new responsibilities. Most of them also did not have the knowledge to deal with the different problems. Yet most of the MWA leaders did not favour the formation of groups among the Indian Muslims. Wherever possible, one or other of its leaders objected and brought to nothing the attempts to organise groups. Only once, after objecting to the formation of a parents' group, did the MWA take over responsibilities for doing what the parents' group had aimed to do. This instance will be discussed later.

The attitude of some of the leaders towards the formation of groups was understandable to some extent. Among some of them there was a genuine fear that if a group was formed for whatever activity, it might one day bring about a split in the Muslim community in Batley. In other words, the Muslims in Batley might one day end up with more than one organisation for seeing to the religious needs of the Muslims. For some of the leaders the reasons for objecting to the formation of groups were different. These men either feared losing their positions or they wanted to be consulted and involved in whatever was going on around them. It seems to me that this response corresponds to the resistance that often comes from existing residents' groups to new developments.

At a later stage in my work, I developed very good contacts with one of the leaders. I started involving him in some of the activities and in this way I was able to reach many other people. I shall discuss this later. Before doing so I shall record the attempts I made to work through groups.

(1) Soon after I joined the project, I found that three men I had come to know wanted to organise a social gathering. I thought the idea worth supporting and acquired the project's backing and a promise for funds to hire a hall. A poets' gathering was held where Indian Muslim poets from Bolton, Preston and Blackburn came to participate. Everything went as planned and about sixty men from the local community turned up. Despite the success, the leaders were not impressed. They felt that the gathering was not in keeping with the community's religious feelings.

(2) During discussions with members of the community, I realised how the communication gap between parents and children was growing. There was a strong feeling that if the children could be taught Gujarati, both the parents and children could communicate better. Six men volunteered to teach Gujarati to the children on Saturdays and Sundays if a school could be found for them. Inquiries were made of the local authority for use of a school building. The plan, however, could not succeed because one of those who had promised to teach thought it proper to seek the permission of the MWA. Without giving any reasons, the MWA decided against the plan to teach, and the idea was dropped.

(3) While the efforts to teach Gujarati were going on, I was also active with the other two project workers in organising a community news-sheet. I knew there was a sizeable number of men in the community who had educational qualifications and I felt that these should be utilised. Again six men showed some interest in the news-sheet. A series of meetings were held to plan it. But when the time came to produce the sheet, only two men remained active. It was later found that out of the four who backed out, two had done so as a result of pressure from some of the leaders. The two remaining men took an active interest and produced two hand-written sheets. After this, a printing press in Preston published the third issue and later on failed to deliver the fourth one. This disheartened the two men who then decided to discontinue the news-sheet.

(4) The MWA became involved in a major way with the local authority in 1976 and this gave me my first and last major chance to work with this organisation. Trouble had come about between Muslim parents and the head of a local girls' high school. The head would not agree to the physical education dress the Muslims were insisting upon for their girls. In order to take up the issue, some fathers had formed themselves into a parents' association. I had helped them do so. But before they had finally formed their association they had asked the MWA to take up the issue with the head teacher and the local authority. At that stage the leaders had declined to do so. Some months later, however, when increasing numbers of parents started approaching the leaders, they decided to take over from the parents' association. My help was sought and, just as I had helped the parents' association, I helped the MWA. Once again, the monopoly position of the MWA became apparent, and the opportunity to initiate new groupings within the community slipped away.

With the involvement of one of the leaders of the MWA who was also a shop steward at one of the mills, I was able to reach a number of men from the community. Through this person I was able to do the following:

(1) I organised meetings with an official of the local authority's education department to discuss the problems of Muslim children at school. These problems usually revolved around school lunches and the clothes the children had to wear at school.
(2) Two meetings were organised with the headmaster of a junior school where 80 per cent of the children were Muslim. This headmaster had insisted that boys wear shorts in his school and the girls wear skirts but not long trousers. This was contrary to the customs and wishes of parents.
(3) Effort was also made to bring the Indian Muslims closer to their ward councillors. A number of meetings were arranged where a group of Muslims could come along to talk with their councillors.
(4) A prospective parliamentary candidate was also introduced to members of the Muslim community enabling him to acquire a better understanding of the community's needs and priorities.
(5) The Indian Muslims were also helped to come closer to the British political system. The leader with whom I was in close contact decided to join a political party, and twenty-three others decided to join along with him.

MY DIFFICULTIES AS A COMMUNITY WORKER

Working with the members of my own ethnic group had advantages and disadvantages. I understood the culture of the people, and as one of them I also understood their problems. Over the period of time I worked with them they came to trust me and confide their problems in me.

Like other community workers I was under constant pressure. As a person who was seen by the community to have education I was supposed to know everything and to be continually resourceful. I think that this high expectation held of me by the community put me at a disadvantage, compared with an English community worker. I could never say 'sorry' or 'no' to the callers. I was expected to deal with whatever problem was brought to me.

Yet despite the trust they had in me and my work, the Indian Muslims did not come to accept me fully as one of them. Though they did not say so, they knew that I worked for a government agency. They also knew that if I was not employed to help them I would not have helped them. As far as they knew, all help had to be paid for, either in cash or in kind, even when it was sought from the members of their own community.

It has been noted already that the indigenous 'advice givers' in Batley who charged for their services were not happy with my presence. To them I meant a loss in their earnings because those who wanted information or filling in of forms came to me. Before I arrived, those who sold their services had a clear field and some of them asked for relatively large sums of money. As a result of this system, people could not understand how they could get free help, except that I was being paid by some organisation to help them. Their experiences in India told them that it was only a government worker or a worker of a government agency who could get things done. For example, they would expect me to telephone the public health inspector about their improvement grants. They believed that the PHI would act swiftly and in a more acceptable manner when requested by me because of my standing as an employee of the CDP. Yet being employed by a government or local government agency also meant that they kept a reserve in certain spheres of their activities. This could be understood if their minority situation and immigrant status was taken into consideration. For example, someone could be, or could have been, an illegal immigrant, or could have been engaged in some illegal activity. It would be expecting too much for an immigrant community to put all its trust in a government-employed worker, particularly for those who knew that the department responsible for the CDP was the Home Office!

There was also an awareness within the community that the CDP was interested in change, and that this might not always be to the advantage of the Muslim Indians. When, therefore, a sensitive religious issue was seen to be at stake, it was natural that someone like myself would not always be very welcome.

To most of the local government officers, trade union officials and others, I was perceived as just another Asian. The only difference was that I worked for a government agency. Over the two-year period in Batley, very few came to identify me as a community worker. Even a community relations officer failed to do so. No amount of argument or explanation could change the preconceived notion of most white people to think otherwise. When, for example, the Housing Action Area was declared, many building contractors were contacted by one of my colleagues in the project. To help overcome the language difficulties I had to accompany these contractors to the Asians' houses. But this did not put me in a position other than being one of the Asians. And with the local government officer this was more or less the same: 'Your people don't keep their gardens tidy', or a similar remark, would clearly identify me with the Asian people and nowhere else as far as I was concerned.

I have indicated some of the difficulties I faced in my work, and I think many of them are shared by other Asian community workers. Yet if an English or non-Muslim community worker had been appointed I am certain that the Indian Muslims would have been left untouched. And without the Gujarati language such a person would have been able to contribute very little.

My involvement in Batley was a consciousness-raising one among the Indian Muslims. I have tried to show how my role kept me on the boundary of the system I worked for and the community I tried to assist. But being a member of the community I was trying to help put me in many instances into the community's territory rather than allowing me to stay on the boundary.

The apparent lack of impact of my community work role on local government, trade union and other agencies reflected, I think, the degree to which I adopted an unfamiliar approach to the Muslim community in my work. I felt I was testing out untried ideas and practice. In retrospect, I was able to see the need to revise many of the theories and strategies favoured by English community workers, as well as my own assumptions about community work. I believe it is important to give Asian workers, and workers of other immigrant cultures, the opportunities to develop effective and relevant approaches to community work, and to ensure an honest sharing of such experiences. This must be the way forward for there to be meaningful community work in immigrant communities.

Chapter 10

COMMUNITY WORK IN BELFAST: A NEIGHBOURHOOD APPROACH

Lisa Huber and Felicity McCartney

This chapter describes the experience of the Centre for Neighbourhood Development, a voluntary agency set up in 1975 to employ and support 'indigenous' community workers to work in neighbourhoods with a population of 3,000 to 6,000 in the Greater Belfast area. By 1978 the centre employed six neighbourhood workers, two support staff and a part-time secretary and had developed a central base as a focus for community work training.

NORTHERN IRELAND

In Northern Ireland before 1969 a situation existed in which the majority of the Catholic population rejected the government, its agencies and allied resources, whilst there was a passive identification by the Protestant community with these institutions. For years there had been little change in the institutions and, with deep divisions in society, there was little demand for growth or the development of new policies. This contributed to the development of serious multiple problems associated with low family income, poor housing conditions, and lack of social amenities. At the same time there existed a wealth of community resources in terms of community care through the extended family and strong community identity.

In these conditions, before and after 1969 community relations deteriorated in the face of civil unrest, intercommunal violence, intimidation and vandalism. 'Institutional violence' also existed, as indicated by the imposition of redevelopment and urban motorway plans, internment, and an inability to provide adequate amenities, social services and employment in many 'working-class' communities. In recent years, in large part a reaction to 'the troubles', there has been a growth of organisations at a local community level concerned with family and community welfare. Parallel to this has been the tendency towards greater centralisation of all the services (housing, health, education, planning) through province-wide agencies and administrative boards.

Through the process of increased awareness of local issues, and organising community action campaigns, more and more people have become involved in their community. They have gained in self-assurance and confidence and have gradually moved on to meet and work with similar people from other areas. Community development can thus provide a bridge for the two communities to meet, as community groups in both Catholic and Protestant communities work on the same problems and issues. Combined action – crossing sectarian divides – on common issues has provided constructive alternatives for the two communities to work together. However, this contact can be exaggerated. A great deal of work still needs to be done at a more local and, therefore, segregated level.

The problems which community groups face in Northern Ireland are similar to those which groups face in other parts of the UK: poor housing, unemployment, transportation plans, changing educational needs, organising effective consultation with government agencies. The violence and civil unrest have contributed to making these social problems worse, as well as making effective action more difficult. The daily violence is fed by these social and economic factors. Thus, the interrelationship between violence and environment must be understood by the community worker.

Conflict in Northern Ireland is usually seen as between Catholic and Protestant communities. However, for the community worker, the more immediate situation is the extent of conflict within the community. This would include the usual conflicts found in all areas – between various interest groups, political groupings, personality clashes and family feuds, as well as loyalties to groups which have emerged through the particular situation in Northern Ireland. Both Catholic and Protestant communities usually have several paramilitary groups, who may have an uneasy alliance, while at other times are in open conflict to secure 'control of the district'. The divisions and animosities between these groups – dividing neighbours as well as families – can be very great. Church groups, political parties and the various peace groups (the Peace People, Women Together, Good Neighbours), also add identifiable factions in the community.

THE PHILOSOPHY OF THE PROJECT

In 1974 a group of fifteen people met to discuss community development, including voluntary and employed community workers, people in the fields of adult education, social work and housing with a strong interest in community development. The group identified support for indigenous neighbourhood work as an important area not developed in Northern Ireland. A British trust agreed to provide a three-year grant for a pilot scheme to employ up to six neighbourhood workers and a support team. Two members of the original group, the authors of this chapter, were employed as support workers in 1975. The project developed a philosophy summarised as follows:

(1) *Intensive community work* in a small neighbourhood allows a fuller understanding of how problems interrelate. Local residents and resources can be involved in solving their problems.
(2) *Indigenous workers,* with experience of community action or voluntary activity, but often without formal qualifications, can be effective and sympathetic community workers given adequate support and training.
(3) The strong *neighbourhood identification* in many areas of Belfast, often manifest negatively through violence, could be positively utilised to enable people to work for social change.
(4) A *support structure* should be developed, each community worker spending half to one day each week in in-service training as part of his job.
(5) A *wider adult education programme* was seen as a natural extension of the centre's support role to help local people to make community action campaigns and activities more effective.

SELECTION OF NEIGHBOURHOODS AND WORKERS

As the project was experimental, an attempt was made to support neighbourhood work in a variety of settings. The communities include neighbourhoods of stable housing, redevelopment areas and new housing estates. The level of community action activity also varied from area to area. It was important that there was some internal support for a community worker in the neighbourhood and this was assessed by the interest and response of individuals and groups in the neighbourhood.

Any community or group could approach the centre for a worker. It was then the responsibility of one of the central support staff to meet with these groups and gain information about the community. This information is brought to the full project committee where the selection of the next project area is made. Once a neighbourhood is selected, the appointment of the worker is a joint venture between the project and the community. Usually the post is widely advertised, and local representatives are included in the shortlisting and interviewing.

This process of consultation is very important, and has had a number of advantages to the development of the neighbourhood work.

(1) Consultation helps to raise the level of understanding about the project's aims and the role of the neighbourhood worker.
(2) It allows time for individuals and groups in the neighbourhood to clarify what they want themselves.
(3) The project staff and committee gained a deeper knowledge and understanding about the neighbourhoods, and were in a better position both to support the neighbourhood worker and to become involved in future decisions about the community.
(4) By consulting other agencies and individuals working in the community the project is able to look at the total neighbourhood and to learn what the other influences on the area are.

THE NEIGHBOURHOOD WORKER AND LOCAL GROUPS

As the neighbourhood workers are indigenous to their communities, local people tend to view them as 'our community worker', in a way in which they would not view other professional community workers. This has both advantages and disadvantages. By coming from the community, the neighbourhood worker usually has local knowledge and relationships within the community which an outside professional would take a very long time to acquire. A disadvantage of a local neighbourhood worker is the amount of pressure put on him or her simply because he or she is from the community and always available. It is also important that the neighbourhood worker tries to remain as neutral as possible in the many conflicts that arise within the neighbourhood. Relationships change in a neighbourhood when a previously voluntary worker becomes paid. Other voluntary workers can feel threatened, demanding or decide to leave everything to the person getting paid. It is the responsibility of the employer to help support their worker through this and to help other local people come to terms with the situation. We have found that the neighbourhood workers have been able to develop the work and gain people's confidence and trust because they live in the area and have many local contacts, and because of the on-going support from the training programme which helps them to see their work in a wider context.

Case Study – Tom

Tom has been working full-time in his neighbourhood for over three years. Before that he was a motor mechanic, but had helped voluntarily for many years with community and youth activities. When he first became the neighbourhood worker he tended to adopt primarily leadership roles. This was natural as he had been chairman or secretary of several community groups. The training programme helped him to identify a number of different roles which he could adopt (facilitator, encourager, trainer) and gradually more and more people were encouraged to take part in community groups and to take over his leadership responsibilities. His comments on his work indicate the importance he placed on working with indivduals: 'People were terrified of joining groups or committees and had to be encouraged'; 'I tried to help bring people out of themselves, people who never thought they were important, to show them that they had knowledge and experience to offer.'

In fact, over the past three years there has been a noticeable increase in the number of people participating in community groups and actively concerned about their district's future. Tom's role has changed primarily to an enabler, where he uses his skill to encourage local involvement and draw in resources. The fact that he already knew so many people has accelerated this process.

This community is literally threatened with its life. All the housing is due for redevelopment and decisions have yet to be made about what land will be used for housing, industry and roads. As it is a Catholic district surrounded by Protestant communities, it has to have adequate land to rehouse enough people within its present boundaries to maintain its schools and church. This crucial situation has given incentive for the groups to organise around housing and planning issues. They are involved in educational work with the community, continuing meetings with the authorities and on developing alternative plans of their own. Tom, who is in contact with all the groups, helps them to arrange programmes and plans, to organise their meetings (often three to four nights a week) and maintain morale. His involvement is steady but he is no longer seen as the leader and works directly with the groups as 'one of them' (his house is coming down too!).

One of the other roles which Tom has played is that of a mediator or go-between. It was important to get all the various groups to work together to avert the threat to the community. For many years conflict within the community could be very destructive. Various political parties, church factions and peace groups would not agree to sit on the same committees but formed their own competing groups. Tom was helpful in encouraging people to work together and to develop housing groups that are representative to the *total* community. This was not easy, but the neutral role he maintained was crucial.

Tom has often been asked to arrange or chair meetings when conflicts arise within the community. This has been a very useful function as intra-community conflict has been very damaging and can quickly escalate in Northern Ireland. He has also been able to act as a liaison between local groups and the security forces, both army and police, when discussions were necessary.

Case Study – Pat

When Pat first started working in her district as a neighbourhood worker it quickly became obvious that many of the residents were concerned about the closure of the local primary school. The district was an old residential area to the north of the city centre, and because of bad housing, rioting and intimidation many families had left the area and the school's population had dropped by two-thirds. The remaining population became totally Protestant who lived in run-down, half-deserted streets, and the school was now situated in a Catholic neighbourhood. This meant providing buses for the short distance (half a mile) or having army patrols supervising the children walking to school. The education authority had decided to close the school but both school staff and parents felt it was a situation that had deteriorated, but could be saved if only they knew what to do and where to go.

Pat began by meeting and discussing the situation with everyone concerned. This included the headmaster, the teachers, the caretaker, parents' association, community groups, the children, local clergy and the education authority. She also visited community groups and the primary school in the neighbouring Catholic district and found they had much the same problems with their school, especially in relation to vandalism. What emerged was a great deal of concern for the school and a lot of positive suggestions to improve the situation. Pat was helpful in bringing the various groups together to discuss the problems, for example, parents with teachers. She helped give people the confidence to express their concerns and their ideas. Nobody involved wanted to see the school closed, an opinion which would not have been expressed publicly without Pat's encouragement.

After several months the education authority reconsidered and reversed their decision, and the school remains open. But, equally important, is that through these meetings a number of growth points, both for community development and improving relations between the two neighbouring communities, emerged, and Pat has used these to further the development work.

Contact between the two primary schools has started in sports and holiday activities. The school is now being used as a base for adult education and a library was organised in a disused classroom. The headmistress has developed a good relationship with Pat and meets with parents in the local community centre. Parents are taking a much more active interest in the school, a change which is welcomed by the teachers. All these developments have contributed to parents and teachers feeling more secure about the school and numbers have been stabilised. Although the Protestant and Catholic neighbourhoods are not mixing yet, Pat keeps in contact with both communities and provides a channel for communication.

Completing and following through a detailed study of this kind takes considerable time and patience. Pat spoke to many people living in and working in the neighbourhoods. These are now contacts which she can develop and use in other ways. As the neighbourhood worker she was accepted by all the groups and was flexible in the roles she adopted, depending on the situation. It is doubtful that a community worker responsible to a large area would have the time or inclination to develop any single project in such depth. But at a neighbourhood level it can be seen how intensive work of this kind can have an ever-expanding effect.

DEVELOPMENT OF THE AGENCY

It has been crucial to the agency that good communication was established between the committee, central office and neighbourhoods. Since its inception, the committee and workers have felt that they must be part of the community development process themselves and be open to ideas and new learning. They often take part in training events along with neighbourhood groups.

Participants in the agency come from a variety of social backgrounds, some motivated by the need to do something positive in a situation of civil conflict or to improve conditions in their own neighbourhood. The group considers working in both Protestant, Catholic and mixed areas – a natural development.

The full participation of all the employed staff (including the office secretary) and representatives from the neighbourhoods in the decision-making in the agency was seen as crucial. A committee including the workers and neighbourhood representatives and 'central' members with skills or interest to contribute was set up for a three-year period. The advantages of this type of committee are that it facilitates communication between the community workers, neighbourhoods, central office and committee members, and helps each to understand the position and outlook of the others. A disadvantage is that the group is large (sixteen to twenty) and increases as new neighbourhoods are added. Some routine business and tasks such as organising conferences, appointment of staff and fund raising have therefore been delegated to broadly based subcommittees or working parties. Discussion of policy and progress remains with the whole committee and care is taken to prepare for these to help informed discussion. For example, each worker writes a full report of his or her work every six months which is considered in some depth at a committee meeting and provides a record of development of the agency and a useful discipline for each worker in planning and evaluating his or her work.

The consensus method of decision-making is used by the group rather than proposing and voting which can be divisive, lead to power blocks and override minority opinion. It requires time, effort and preparation to inform each member about each issue. The role of the chairperson is changed in that there is no casting vote, though he or she still has the responsibility to distil the discussion and help the group to arrive at a decision. The officers have changed twice in the first three years allowing more people to take on responsibility. The agency's commitment to consensus and participation means that it cannot be allowed to grow much bigger than twenty people. Further increase in this work could be facilitated by encouraging other similar centres to grow, with their own autonomy and a fraternal relationship to this centre.

The commitment to provide adequate support and in-service training was to help people to be more effective in their roles as community worker, local activist or committee member. In practice, the two community workers in the central office were appointed first and given the responsibility to develop training and support for the project members and education activities for the community in general (for example, to enable local groups to gain expertise in running a community centre, redevelopment, young children, welfare rights). These courses were organised both locally – held in the community centre – and centrally, giving an opportunity for community groups from different areas to meet and share experiences. For the neighbourhood workers a flexible pattern of in-service training emerged which, with regular modification, has been followed. The project committee felt that it was important to create and maintain conditions favourable to their employment so that a full-time position could be seen as a long-term commitment. This continuity is especially important at a neighbourhood level and the continued support given to the workers is an important factor in their ability to maintain interest and enthusiasm for the job.

Initial Period (1–2 months)

When community workers are first appointed they are usually enthusiastic to organise projects. They are under pressure from the local community to justify their job and may be unrealistic about the time needed to produce 'results'. There is a body of skills and information which they will need in order to assess each neighbourhood's problems and their role in helping to solve them.

An induction programme is organised by the centre during this time. Most of the content is planned for the new worker but the whole staff group helps to plan and join in about one-third of the

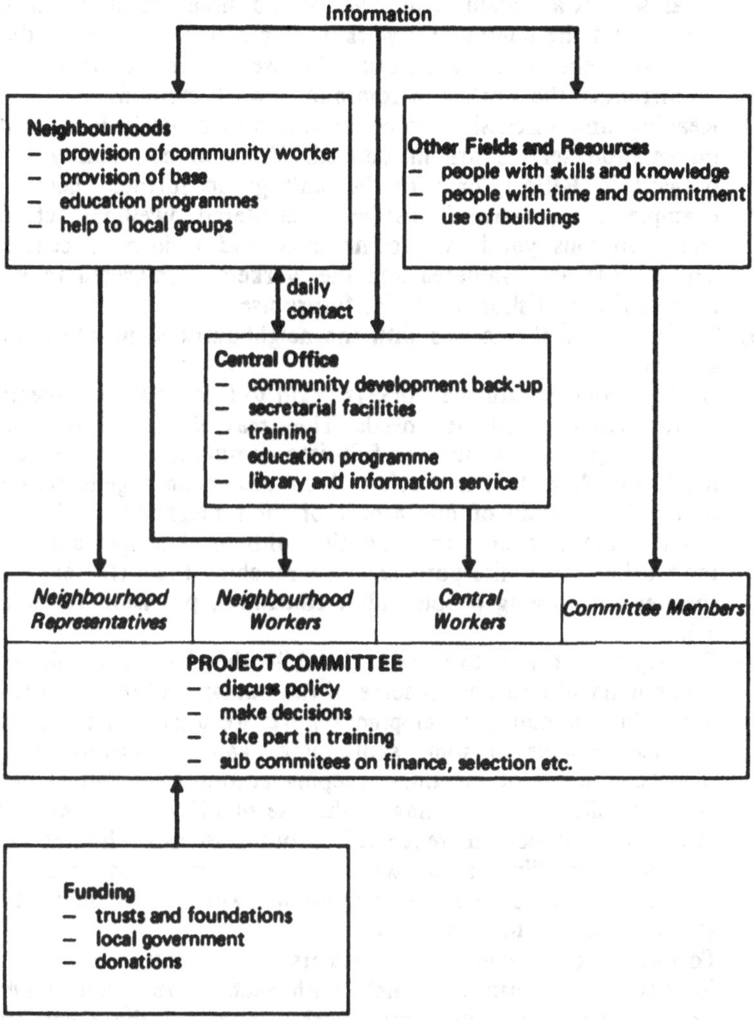

Figure 10.1. *Diagram Showing Relationships and Activities in the Centre for Neighbourhood Development.*

sessions. The programme occupies each day for three to four weeks and approximately two days a week for a further month. The aims and content can be summarised as follows:

(1) To familiarise the new worker with agencies and resources. A programme of visits to local offices of social service, housing, youth, social security departments, etc., and to relevant voluntary

organisations are planned in advance and discussed fully with the agency and the community worker. Evaluation sessions on these visits are held to help the worker to assess their usefulness.

(2) To introduce the worker to community work methods.
Reading and discussion based around the centre's library and information service are introduced. Visits to community work projects in Belfast, or with the staff group further afield (for example, co-operative industries, a sheltered dwellings scheme, and numerous youth and community and residential centres). These visits are evaluated and the workers encouraged to keep address lists and short notes for future use.

(3) To familiarise themselves with the neighbourhood in which they will work.
In the second month the workers begin to look at their respective neighbourhoods and their needs. They may already be part of it but their role will change as full-time community workers. They need to explain their new role to local groups and agencies. They undertake a study of one aspect of their neighbourhood which requires them to take the initiative with local people and gives the workers a definite purpose in approaching them (for example, the needs of young people, adult education, provision for under 5s).

(4) To help the workers to identify the skills they have and will need.
Preliminary discussions on some of the human and technical skills useful in community development work are organised along with practice sessions in some skills. For example, writing letters, reports, minutes of meetings, keeping accounts, are all included and are followed by training in the use of office equipment, film projectors and video as requested. Group sessions on human skills such as counselling, group work and basic psychology are occasionally organised and the community workers encouraged to attend outside courses on these.

(5) To introduce the community workers to the centre.
Introductory meetings are held with each of the central office workers, with the community work group and the committee, and background reading is done, often before the worker is actually in post.

First Year

After the initial few months the workers can take on a few limited projects, preferably along with local groups, and they are more confident that they have something to offer. They will probably have a landslide of requests, many inappropriate, from people with problems they expect them to solve.

During this period, the individual support session becomes more important and is held between community worker and a central worker each week for up to two hours. The workers begin to sort out their priorities in relation to local needs and pressures, their own abilities and available resources. They may have to work through an initial instinct to do everything for people to a position where they encourage people's own initiative, local groups and appropriate agencies to help.

Group sessions continue once or twice monthly and allow community workers to share experience. Outside speakers are often asked, for example, a lawyer, officials from government departments and members of community groups with expertise in particular fields (supplementary benefits, play, housing). About one day per week is now spent on training and central activities.

Second Year

By the second year, community workers have a much clearer idea of what initiatives they should take. The individual sessions can be used more for self-evaluation. They can identify what they want to achieve more clearly: 'How can I help this group organise a youth club (housing campaign, advice centre, etc.)?'; 'How will I react to a local leader (official, voluntary worker) with whom I can't agree?'. The workers can articulate their own training needs more clearly as they become secure enough to say; 'I am good at this but not at that', and often group sessions are organised on this analysis and less initiative taken by the central workers.

THE FUTURE

The project has now come to the end of its initial period of three years. From the start, with three workers, the staff has gradually increased to the full team of six neighbourhood workers, two support staff, and a secretary. The committee has developed into a strong, confident group. After three years of raising all its own budget, the project has recently been approved for government grant aid (approximately 60 per cent). Our financial and structural independence through the formative years were crucial to developing the community work programme. There is now a growing awareness within the project that there should be an attempt to communicate our experience and to take a more active role in influencing other agencies and groups.

Major decisions and the allocating of resources which affect people most are not taken at a community level. Thus the community work strategy must work upwards as well as outwards. It is quite possible to effect development within a neighbourhood and to have helpful relationships with agency staff without having any basic effect on the agency centrally or its policy and practices. To influence the agencies centrally is a job for all the community workers and for the project as a whole. It is hoped to assess common problems and practices from the different neighbourhoods and for the project as an agency with considerable contact and experience of many communities in Belfast, to stimulate discussion, and organise effective strategies, thereby complementing the in-depth work at a neighbourhood level.

PART THREE

INFLUENCE, ORGANISATION AND PROFESSIONAL GROWTH

INTRODUCTION

There is a sense in which the shift from reading case studies of community work practice to examining the content of this final section mirrors the feelings many community workers have when they compare their work in neighbourhoods or on issues with work inside or between bureaucratic organisations. The former inspires total commitment and a sense that 'this is what community work is all about'. The latter, if it is not frowned upon as a hybrid form of community work, lacks the equivalent promise of exhilaration.

Discussion of the degree to which community work has influenced a number of disciplines and organisations, an assessment of its organisational context, and thirdly, analysis of the debate about professionalisation and social movements, are designed to counter the above doubts. If there is substance in our opinion that community work has developed in this country largely on the boundaries of existing organisations, and that energies have not been directed to building up community work as a distinctive method of intervention, then examination of the above topics must be sustained. Debate about community work and organisations, and about professionalisation, far from being *passé*, could benefit from greater incisiveness. Even concern about the opportunities, constraints and conditions of service at their places of work has been neglected by community workers until quite recently. It does not compare, for example, with the time and energy concentrated on the question of training.

It is likely that the folly of ignoring organisational and professional issues will become more apparent as the extent to which community work is lodged in the public sector becomes more obvious. The latter development is implicit in Brian Munday's assessment of community work's influence on the social work and health professions in Chapter 11. It forms a central part of Chapter 12 by Phil Doran, and in Chapter 13 Teresa Smith also pinpoints (from Specht's analysis) community workers' mistrust of the public sector, both as employer and as a major source of resources and services.

The ways in which community work has permeated other disciplines give Brian Munday the opportunity to range widely and, in doing so, to indicate common features in different settings. He maintains, for example, that 'Christian community workers employed by churches often experience similar conflicts to those faced by community workers in social services departments'. He also indicates what kind of contribution community work can bring to 'political responsibilities and powers accompanying any professional work carried out under the auspices of government'. This surely suggests one of the positive features arising from community work's engagement with related disciplines, organisations and professions.

We state in the Introduction that the question of who employs the community worker is a crucial one in relation to interjacence. Phil Doran approaches it primarily by examining his own community work experience in relation to employing organisations and to central government policies, and by advancing clear opinions. It is interesting to set his views alongside the considerable American research and writing on the same subject – the section on sponsorship in George Brager and Harry Specht's book *Community Organising* (New York: Columbia University Press, 1973), for example, and Ralph Kramer's 'The influence of sponsorship, professionalism and the civic culture on the theory and practice of community development' in the second edition of R. Kramer and H. Specht's *Reading in Community Organisation Practice* (Englewood Cliffs, N.J.: Prentice-Hall, 1975). Doran refers to local authorities as bureaucratic systems and contends that 'any mature system, especially a democratic system, must build into itself a self-critical mechanism'. He argues in favour of local authority community workers, and urges them to make more skilled use of their employment bases: 'Too often community workers in local authorities are unaware of how decisions are made and of the relationships necessary to achieve results.'

The final contribution appropriately brings us back to such fundamental questions as, where do community workers get their legitimacy from? Is the social movement tradition the only one capable of handling the essentially political nature of the issues in community work? Teresa Smith points out that, despite the debate which has been pursued, there is still little agreement on whether community work is or should be considered a profession. By examination of relevant literature she offers a way forward by evaluating both sides of the argument and searching for a synthesis: 'Community work can be seen as a profession to which protest movements have made considerable contributions.'

Close analysis of the concepts of profession and social movement, not allowing them to retain their ambiguities, suggests how easy it might be to misinterpret our discussion of the boundary role of community work. It is one thing to function as an interjacent activity, quite another to fail to survive. Community work can ill afford, at this point in time, not to attend to questions relating to organisational analysis and professionalisation, with rigour and imagination. The development of community work as an effective form of intervention would seem to depend as much upon this as upon continuing experience and evaluation of practice. Together they can inject an essential dynamic element into community work practice and theory. We take up this point in the concluding chapter.

Chapter 11

THE PERMEATION OF COMMUNITY WORK INTO OTHER DISCIPLINES

Brian Munday

The purpose of this chapter is to discuss the nature and extent of the permeation of community work into related disciplines and services, with special reference to social work and the personal social services (PSS), medicine and the health services, and the Christian ministry and the church.

Both Gulbenkian reports on community work (Gulbenkian Foundation, 1968, 1973) referred at length to the need for community work to influence the development of a wide range of related activities, particularly through training. The first report supported the view that as well as being a full-time professional task, community work should also be conceived and practised as a function exercised by many different people as part of their professional or voluntary activities. The Maud (1967) and Mallaby (1967) reports are quoted approvingly with their reference to the importance of both councillors and officials in local government gaining a thorough understanding of the community perspective. There was a recommendation that all local authority officers should have, as part of their training, a substantial area of common study of the social conditions in which they operate. The first Gulbenkian report goes on to refer to 'technical man as community worker', technical man being town clerks, doctors, education officers, physical planners, social workers and their like. At the senior level these people, who are found within the power structures of society with considerable responsibility for planning and administration of services, need training to understand the community perspective of their posts. This report was very influential in advocating that the values, objectives, knowledge and methods of community work as a slowly developing discipline should permeate a number of related activities, to the ultimate benefit of the community.

Five years later the second Gulbenkian report was enthusiastic about the degree to which this permeation by community work had taken place, particularly as judged by developments in training for related professional groups. The report stated that it was 'clear that many more administrative and professional groups are taking account of what they consider to be the social dimension of their work'. Recent developments in curricula of medical and para-medical training, as well as training for planners and architects, all indicated a growing recognition to understand more about the communities with which these professions are involved. The report cites evidence from a survey to show the increase in the community work content in social work courses from 1967 to 1972, a development that will be considered in more detail later. The report writers agreed that their results were impressionistic but they referred to a 'dramatic increase' of other professions' perception of the direct relevance of an articulate understanding of community processes and other key community work concepts and concerns, including the fundamental principle of consultation with the people concerned about decisions which affect their lives.

More specifically, there was evidence of a gradual introduction into courses for planners and architects of knowledge about communities and of community work as a method of work in neighbourhoods. In medical education there had been a noticeable increase in teaching of the behavioural sciences, including sociology, and more emphasis on social factors related to medicine. Similar trends were evident in the training of health visitors. In a variety of ways teacher training courses were seen to be trying to give students an insight into the complexities of community life, with the school as one of the institutions concerned with improvements in the quality of life. In 1972, Ilkley College in Yorkshire started a three-year course in community education, designed to give teachers experience of community needs and problems. Students working in Educational Priority Area schools were able to take part in community work projects, school-based or otherwise. Similar trends were reported in the training of young administrators in central government; the clergy; lawyers with the extension of legal services to the more deprived sections of the community through neighbourhood law centres; and the police with special emphasis on community and race relations work.

Following this chronicle of impressive success by community work in infiltrating other disciplines through training content, the report goes on to advocate that the study of community structure, relations and changing patterns should be taught at appropriate levels during school years to help children develop an intelligent understanding of our changing society. This theoretical study could be related to voluntary community service in local areas, an activity that has certainly developed rapidly since 1973.

To claim that community work has permeated all manner of related services and professions implies that some of community work's values, objectives, knowledge, skills and methods have somehow diffused or penetrated into these other activities and helped to shape their identity and purpose. This sounds a grandiose claim for community work to make, particularly if a cause–effect relationship is being argued. The explanation of the apparent espousal of community work by other disciplines is more complex than a simple causal link from community work to the other disciplines. For example, the admittedly limited interest in client and citizen participation in the personal social services can be attributed more to a growing movement throughout our society for consumer rights and participation, than to the direct influence of community work with its traditional emphasis on participation. It is now acknowledged that the official services with their armies of professionals can never cope with the totality of demand for social and health care, even if it was desirable that they should do so. Hence the increasing interest in the contribution of a range of non-agency community personnel to the provision of social care, epitomised in the work of the Volunteer Centre with its current emphasis on neighbour care. There are signs here of a more sophisticated approach to the theory and practice of community care which will look to community work for insights and methods.

My view is that an increasing number of professions and services now share some of the basic tenets of community work, but this is not to argue that this phenomenon has resulted from missionary zeal by community work. A discipline will make use of concepts and methods from another discipline for its own purposes without being invited to do so. For example, in the 1960s and 1970s 'community' became something of a bandwagon term, applied often indiscriminately to jobs and services in other disciplines to give a progressive, modern image, as well as indicating a policy shift from care in institutions to care in the community. It certainly does not necessarily mean that the spirit and practice of community work has been incorporated into the other disciplines. Professions will often share knowledge, values and practice skills which do not result from the direct influence or permeation of one by the other.

Rather than adopt a missionary outlook, many community workers are fearful of the close involvement with other services and professions which is needed if some of the basic values, knowledge and methods of community work are to penetrate into related activities. As Thomas and Warburton (1977) show in their study of community workers in a social services department, community workers are ever alive to the danger of 'going native', fearing that they will be incorporated into the other agency or professional group. In Chapter 5 above, Poulton refers to the related concept of 'frontiersman', the moving into uncharted territory to study and possibly colonise the natives. Poulton sees this as a concept that hovers uneasily around community development in industrialised countries. Community workers might feel more secure in a frontiersman role if they were more certain of the distinctive contribution of their own discipline – a useful protection against the danger of 'going native'.

The extent to which community work is able to permeate related activities will depend heavily upon resolution of a central paradox. Assuming that community workers do want to contribute to the development and identity of other professions and organisations, they need to be reasonably sure of the identity of their own discipline, particularly its theory and methods of practice. A constant tension for community work has been the need to look inwards to the building up of the knowledge and skills base of the discipline, as well as looking outwards to influence other disciplines. This has created a tension by no means peculiar to community work. But, as this book demonstrates, there are characteristics of community work which leave it ill equipped to permeate extensively other activities and professions. For example, community work is described in the Introduction to this book as a 'marginal activity in our society, marginal in relation to major political, economic and social welfare institutions and forces'. In her critique of the place of community work in local government, Cockburn (1977) refers to community workers as 'corporate agents operating at the periphery of the system, organising corporate behaviour in the community, encouraging community oriented behaviour in the local state and fixing up interaction between the two'. Thomas and Warburton and other writers have shown how community work tends to operate on the boundary, clarifying the structural relationship of the community worker in relation to his or her community groups, and employing agency, and his or her occupation in relation to others such as social work, planning and adult education.

The effectiveness of community work must rest partly on the outsider role of the community worker, as incorporation into a related discipline would distort the special contribution of community work. It remains to be seen whether the marginal man can make a real impact outside his own discipline if the tendency continues towards larger service organisations and the proliferation of separate professional groups. Community workers of the exogenous type described by Thomas and Warburton (1977) are at great pains to carve out and protect a boundary role in relation to both social work and their employing departments. They neither seek nor achieve a permeation of community work attributes into these two related systems, though this permeation may still take place under other influences.

THE INFLUENCE OF COMMUNITY WORK ON SOCIAL WORK AND THE PERSONAL SOCIAL SERVICES

Social Work

There are good reasons for believing that community work has permeated social work more extensively than any other activity. Unlike the situation in the USA where community organisation has developed within social work, in Britain there is a different tradition and a greater degree of separation. In this process some community workers have portrayed a distorted stereotype of social work as inherently conservative, using a psycho-dynamic form of repressive casework to fit victims of our unjust economic and social system back into that same system.

There are several reasons for believing that community work has substantially permeated social work and the PSS. First, there have been important developments in social work training, which I discuss later. Secondly, a large number of community workers are employed in social services departments, many of these community workers with training and experience in social work. Other evidence is found in the growing interest in assessing needs and. resources in social services departments and in the decentralisation of services, for example through patch systems of working. Institutional opportunities exist for community work to influence the PSS and social work through representation of the community work interest in the Central Council for Education and Training in Social Work, the British Association of Social Workers and the Personal Social Services Council. It would be difficult to assess how well these opportunities are used. Tasker and Wunnam (1977) credit community work with a very significant influence upon British social work. In their article they claim that 'Social work has been heavily influenced recently by two radical trains of thought . . . One is the growth of the community development movement which has been partly in alliance with social work and partly separate.' The other radical influence on social work they see as a radical political movement within social work itself. The writers conclude that enormous benefit has accrued to social work from the stimuli of these two developments.

The particular contribution of community work has been to emphasise the social rather than the individual dimension in discussion of personal distress and social problems, since in their interpretations of social malaise community workers are more likely than social workers to proffer social, political and economic dimensions to explanations of social problems. Community work has also drawn attention to political responsibilities and powers accompanying any professional work carried out under the auspices of government. Tasker and Wunnam even go so far as to claim for community work that 'The radical movements have encouraged in social work the acceptance of a general outgoing toughness as not simply an acceptable but a *necessary* personality characteristic in a profession where once a capacity for introspection and a gentle compassion could suffice and indeed prevailed' (my emphasis).

It is very difficult to be certain about how radical or otherwise any profession may be and how or why a profession may have become more radical than it was in the past. Social work is more politically radical now than in the early 1960s, in that more social workers acknowledge the root economic and political causes of individual clients' problems and are prepared to advocate and work for solutions that entail changing systems outside the identified client. Assuming this is so, there have been radicalising influences on social work in addition to and perhaps more powerful than that of community work. There were, for example, many young people coming into social work training and practice in the early 1970s who had been radicalised politically as students during the peak of left-wing politics on the campuses in the late 1960s and early 1970s. On graduation a proportion of these young people turned to jobs in community work or social work as a way of giving expression to their radical beliefs. A related radical influence on social work has been a politically leftward shift in the teaching of the social sciences on many social science courses.

I see community work as an important but only one of several radicalising influences on social work. The actual permeation of social work by community work (by no means always a politically radical influence) has taken place chiefly through training. Earlier in this chapter I referred to the evidence in the second Gulbenkian report of a considerable increase in the teaching of community work on social work courses from 1967–72, a trend which I am sure has continued and been developed in ways which I shall discuss. But it is not only at the basic training level that social workers are taught and gain practice experience in community work. For some years the National Institute for Social Work has taught community work at the post-qualification level for social workers and Aberdeen University now offers a CCETSW-approved, post-qualification course in community work for experienced social workers. Social workers are able to train on part-time, sandwich community work courses in other institutions, as well as learn more of community work and its application to social work through agency-based, in-service programmes. But I wish to focus mainly on the teaching of community work on qualifying courses in social work, as it is here that community work has achieved a significant permeation of social work, a mixture of both cause and effect of the two disciplines moving closer together, with more of the movement coming from social work.

It is impossible to generalise about all social work courses but I think it possible to talk of a discernible tendency. The most significant training development in my view has not been the sheer quantitative increase in some definable community work content in the syllabi of social work courses, but rather in the way in which much of this content has slowly moved in from a precarious position on the periphery of the courses to acceptance as part of the mainstream teaching. In doing so, some of the previously labelled 'community work syllabus' has been renamed and its distinctive, rather separate community work identity forgotten. I realise this is by no means the case with all courses, but I think developments on my own course are sufficiently typical to warrant discussion.

In the early 1970s a short sequence on community work was included in the two-year syllabus of our two-year graduate course, partly because of student demand and partly because this was seen as a relatively new, interesting field of practice that social work students should know about. A small number of students experienced community work in a fieldwork placement, seen as a somewhat suspect activity on a social work training course. From that beginning, the basic teaching for all students on 'What is community work?' increased in quantity, as did the number of community work placements, to be followed later by an option course on community work which appealed strongly to students who were beginning to suspect that for them community rather than social work would be more suitable. By now the community work content of the two-year programme had increased substantially but it was still seen as a relatively marginal part of the course. At this point the formulations of Pincus and Minahan (1973) and Goldstein (1973) helped us to recognise more forcibly that there was a substantial common area of values, knowledge and methods shared by community work and the kind of social work needed in the 1970s. Instead of teaching all students about community work as an important but separate activity, we have designed a core course containing practice knowledge and skills that are common to both community work and social work. The second-year community work option course has been retained, but is of interest increasingly to students who want to stay in social work but extend the range of methods they can use to deal with community needs and problems, rather than using this course as part of the escape to what has been seen as the more radical community work.

I am not saying that community work and social work are the same but, on our course and many others, a good deal of the theoretical and practice teaching previously seen as special to community work has gradually been drawn into the main stream of the course and has helped to bring about an expanded understanding of the purpose, knowledge and methods of social work. Examples of the theoretical and practice teaching are seminars on community needs and resources; influencing organisations; and working with community groups. Therefore, I argue that to varying degrees the values, knowledge and methods of community work (for fuller details see, for example, Association of Community Workers, 1975) have been incorporated into social work at the basic training level. What difference that makes to the subsequent practice of the social workers is another matter.

The Personal Social Services

Despite these changes in the training and outlook of many social workers, their chief employers – social services departments – have been slow to develop the community-oriented approach so strongly advocated in chapter 16 of the Seebohm Report (1968).

The Seebohm recommendations are well known. The Committee advocated a wider conception of social service directed to the well-being of the whole of the community and seeing the community it serves as the basis for its authority, resources and effectiveness. The PSS should engage in encouraging and assisting the development of community identity and mutual aid, particularly in high-social-need areas. Community development work was needed 'to help the spontaneous development of neighbourhood interests and activities in meeting needs'. Wider groups in society would need help to perform many of their mutual aid and caring functions, in the same way that families needed this help from statutory and voluntary services. The importance of citizen participation is a principal value and objective of community work and it was strongly urged upon social services departments by Seebohm. The rationale for this was recognition that in the PSS the consumer has limited choice among services and needs special opportunities to participate. He or she lacks the consumer's most compelling sanction against a supplier. Very importantly, citizen participation should reduce the distinction between givers and receivers, and the stigma so often involved in being a client.

Because of its centrality in community work it is worth inquiring how far this principle of participation – with all its acknowledged shortcomings (see Arnstein, 1969) – has been accepted and implemented in the PSS. According to Leigh (1977) this participation has failed to gain a strong foothold in social services departments. He identified three kinds of participation in the planning of local social services:

(1) The inclusion of consumers and some kinds of service providers (e.g. foster parents) in the decision-making process. One method would be to co-opt such people on to social services' committees.
(2) Active consultation with consumers and voluntary groups about how services should develop.
(3) Various groups taking a critical, pressure-group role *vis-à-vis* the PSS.

There are examples of departments co-opting consumer representatives on to social services' committees and, at the practice end, of attempts to give the elderly a say in how old people's homes are run; but Leigh concludes that so far in Britain there has been very little attempt to enable outsiders to participate in the decision-making process. Interestingly, in the USA several states make a statutory requirement on agencies to provide means of citizen participation in the planning of social services. In this country, resistance to participation comes both from staff in social services departments and from councillors. The former see it as enormously time-consuming and a threat to their professional position, while councillors are traditionally suspicious of pressure groups and view participation as potentially a conflict-creating process. Sadly, Specht (1974) found in interviews with a considerable number of British community workers that though many were keenly committed to the principle of citizen participation, none had considered how to structure the participation of consumers into the decision-making system of their departments. This criticism leads me to the final comment on community work's impact on social services departments.

With 251 community workers employed (according to the DHSS) by social services departments in 1975 and an even larger number now, it seems reasonable to expect a noticeable permeation of community work principles and methods into the work of the departments through the influence of these workers. They might be expected to act as agents influencing the social work-dominated institutions more and more towards community work approaches. A simple example would be where a community worker encourages a social services' team to look for common problems evident in individuals' caseloads. A crop of complaints about lack of play facilities for young children could result in a community worker and social workers helping parents to organise and take collective action. Without a community worker's encouragement and expertise social workers may not adopt this collective approach.

Community workers might well criticise this expectation as unrealistic, for reasons such as the heavy statutory responsibility of departments for individual cases, and because community workers are spread very thinly through the many departments. I accept the partial validity of these and other arguments. Nevertheless, impressionistic evidence, plus empirical evidence from the Thomas and Warburton study (1977), indicate that a significant number of community workers in social services departments have no interest in influencing thinking, attitudes and practice within their organisations, and aggressively keep their distance from all non-community work staff. I regard this approach as counter-productive for the cause of community work, while appreciating the dangers for community workers of being colonised and pressed into undertaking quite inappropriate work. In Chapter 6 above, O'Hagan's account of his work in Camden shows the value of the integration of community work with other aspects of a department's work.

In the study of eleven community workers and their supervisors in one social services department, Thomas and Warburton (1977) refer to the group of exogenous workers. These workers are likely to distinguish sharply between agency and community work and confine themselves to direct work with neighbourhood groups. They did not accept an educational role in respect of other staff in the department. In contrast with another group of community workers in the department who tried to act as change-agents in the organisation and seek views of social workers on possible new projects determined by community needs, the exogenous workers feared the direction of their work by non-community workers if they became too involved with other staff. One such community worker said: 'I don't approve of the idea that I'm placed in an area team and I don't intend to make that anything more than a formality, if possible . . . I'm not trying to be nasty but I would hope there wouldn't be too much contact with social workers . . . I don't see my job as part of their set up . . .'

Thomas and Warburton rightly claim that there has been too much concentration on problems and constraints and too little on advantages and opportunities of community work in social services departments. They mention two features of departments that provide opportunities for community workers to exploit. First, the tendency for global objective statements that provide sanction for a wide range of activities by astute community workers. Secondly, the recognition that social services departments are not organisations with simple and uncontroversial goals. There are contradictions which can be exploited by community workers who can make a contribution to goal-setting within the organisation. I would add two other features that need exploitation by community workers. First, the existence of many social workers who will look to community workers for help in extending their own range of methods of work with community needs and problems, rather than crudely seeking to convert community workers into caseworkers. Secondly, the rapidly growing interest in new-style community and neighbourhood care to which community workers will be expected to make a significant theoretical and practice contribution. In my view, there remains an enormous potential for non-compromised community work in social services departments that has yet to be taken up.

MEDICINE AND HEALTH CARE

I argue in this section that medicine and the health services remain far more impervious to and less in sympathy with community work values and methods than has been the case with social work and the PSS. The introduction of terms like community medicine, community physician and community health councils (CHCs) in no way means that Illich (1975) and other radical critics of medicine have been taken note of, with general practitioners turned into community health workers and patient power predominating over traditional élites in the National Health Service (NHS). On the whole, doctors continue to be preoccupied with the functioning of individual bodies, while doctors and the post-reorganisation bureaucrats are overwhelmingly the power holders in the NHS.

Western medicine now seems too narrowly concerned with individual patients, at the expense of health and illness promoting factors in the wider community. This has not always been the case. Fraser (1973) argues that in the first half of the nineteenth century doctors became increasingly aware of the health implications of urban life and 'did more to improve the nation's health by identifying the public health problems . . . than by any improved techniques in the treatment of patients'. Chadwick's *Report of the Sanitary Conditions of the Labouring Population of Great Britain* (1842) established the incontrovertible link between environment and disease. Despite much political and ideological opposition, Chadwick's work contributed signficantly to the Public Health Act of 1948, a great landmark in social reform. Although mortality rates in all social classes have fallen substantially, rates are still disproportionately high in the lower social classes. Individually oriented Western doctors remain insufficiently concerned about possible causes and remedies for this disturbing phenomenon.

Until quite recently, community workers in Britain had also largely neglected health issues. This has been partly because, with the exception of health education officers, the health authorities have not employed staff with a brief to concentrate on environmental factors related to ill health. In Sydney, Australia, I was interested to find multi-disciplinary community health centres set up by the Health

Commission with community workers employed to tackle 'unhealthy' environmental factors such as housing.

In Britain, there are signs that community workers, together with neighbourhood and interest groups, are now beginning to work on health issues and to campaign against the inadequacies of the NHS. The Albany Neighbourhood Health Project in south-east London is a good example of this development in community work. This project arose because of the obvious gaps in the NHS, including a lack of preventive work, plus a widespread feeling of powerlessness by local residents when faced with clinicians. The project will work with various self-help groups concerned with the prevention of ill health and collaborate with tenants' associations and trades councils in tackling environmental health issues. A fundamental principle of the project is that local residents should be involved to the maximum.

If we take the broader view of health services, namely health care which encompasses official and all manner of voluntary and informal health caring in society, then we find developments which are much more in sympathy with the spirit and practice of community work. Outside the NHS, we are witnessing the growth of a vigorous self-help movement with a burgeoning of groups of fellow-sufferers (see Robinson and Henry, 1977) who are concerned with prevention as well as amelioration of ill health, who work from participatory principles, and at times act as local and national pressure groups. Community workers tend to be suspicious of any enthusiasm for self-help because of its nineteenth-century conservative connotations, but it now covers a wide range of ideologies and in the health care field represents the community-based and oriented end of a continuum of health service provision. However, for the rest of this section I propose to concentrate on the official health services and consider to what extent the introduction of the various 'community' terms indicates that medicine and the NHS are being influenced by the spirit and practice of community work.

Community Health Councils

These were set up under the reorganisation of the NHS in 1974 to provide a new way of representing the local community's interest in the health service, with one CHC for each health district. Each CHC has eighteen to thirty members, one-third appointed by local authorities, one-third by the regional health authority and one-third by voluntary organisations. The regional health authority nominees are supposed to ensure that there is a fair balance of local interests, for example there has to be a representative of a local trades council. A critical consideration is to what extent a cross-section of local interests are represented on CHCs. Almost certainly Wandsworth local authority is atypical in giving all their nominations to 'grass-roots' organisations.

The CHCs have three main functions: to deal with complaints, to contest closure of services, and to improve services.

Ham (1977) sees CHCs faced with the central problem of what role to adopt in their relationships with the health authorities. He bluntly comments that if they are patients' watchdogs then they become either 'snivelling lap dogs or rabid curs'. Many CHCs have taken a middle line and become a 'critical friend'. The majority have undoubtedly tended towards the consensual end of the role spectrum, and been far too polite and deferential. They can act to widen public debate on health and press for improvements in service but they can too easily provide a smokescreen of public participation in the run-down of service. There are examples of CHCs acting in a more aggressive, campaigning way. South Camden CHC provided information and support to workers occupying the Elizabeth Garrett Anderson Hospital in London to retain it as a women's hospital. Similarly, Wandsworth and East Merton CHC provided a valuable information service to a campaign fighting to save the closure of a small maternity hospital. Delegates from several CHCs took part in a day of action in November 1976 to protest about the deliberate policy of running-down London's health services. Despite the obvious structural weakness of the CHCs in the NHS system, community groups do need to fight to make them represent their interests. Close collaboration between CHCs and local voluntary and community groups is crucial if a 'health consciousness' is to be developed and become as vital an issue as race and housing.

Community Medicine and the Community Physician

The short publication by the Faculty of Community Medicine (1977) provides a good account of the discipline and the practitioner. In a different publication, Dr Arie (1975), a Fellow of the Faculty, is very critical of medicine's jump on to the community bandwagon. He complains that 'Community medicine now leads the field, perhaps exploiting the cosy idea of "Community" in common with a growing brood of disparate siblings: community care, community hospitals etc.'. Both community medicine and the community physician are developments from the reorganised NHS. Community medicine is concerned with the assessment of a community's health needs and with the provision of services to communities in general and to special groups in them. It is concerned with the demography of an area and with relating health and illness there to questions of class, ethnic composition and similar factors. Knowledge of the occurrence of health and illness in the local population indicates what action needs to be taken, for example health education and social policies aimed at modifying illness-provoking behaviour.

The community physician has to practise community as opposed to clinical medicine in his area. He is charged with the health of a particular population and responsible for linking health with other services such as education and the PSS. Arie (1975) underlines the enormous potential of the role of the community physician in helping to further the health interests of all groups in the community: 'The community doctor's commitment to objective appraisal gives him an obvious role as advocate for the under-privileged, the medically unprestigious and the politically inarticulate.' He could be a powerful ally of community groups and community workers but this potential is only very partially realised. His role in the NHS is an uncertain one and devalued by many consultants and administrators who consider the job could be done by a layman. There is still the notion abroad in medicine that you are not a proper doctor if you are not treating patients. Small wonder that there is a lack of recruits for these posts, with a hundred vacancies at any one time.

Medical Training and Education

I argued earlier that community work's permeation of social work has been achieved chiefly through changes in the content of training where community work values, knowledge and skills are being selectively integrated into the core teaching on social work courses. If doctors are to gain greater understanding of social, economic and political factors related to health and illness, and adapt their practice accordingly, then there must be changes in their education and training similar to those evident in social work. After all, the greatest improvements in health have resulted from improvements in social and environmental conditions rather than from improvements in medical treatment of individuals.

One quantifiable change that should gradually help to change doctors' understanding and attitudes has been the increase in the teaching of the behavioural sciences in undergraduate medical courses. The *Report of the Royal Commission on Medical Education* (Todd Report, 1968) quotes the General Medical Council's recommendation that 'In the undergraduate medical course instruction should be given in those aspects of the behavioural sciences which are relevant to the study of man as an organism adapting to his social and psychological, no less than to his physical environment.' Medical education was seen as in need of great improvement in teaching doctors to understand patients as people whose difficulties are often social in origin. For example, by 1968 few medical schools offered any organised teaching in sociology. The Report recommended that sociologists, social administrators and social workers all might contribute to the teaching of the social dimensions of medicine. I would like to think that as more community workers gain experience of work with health issues they, too, will make a contribution to medical education at all levels.

In her survey of the teaching of sociology in medical schools, Maclean (1975) found a wide variation in curricular time from nought to ninety hours, with differing selections of subjects to teach under this heading. As from 1974, the University of London obliged their schools of medicine to include sociology as applied to medicine during part II of the MB, BS course. Among the sociology subjects that should be related to health, illness and the health services were social class, ethnicity, kinship, urbanisation, stigma, employment, bureaucracy and professionalism. As for the actual implementation of this kind of teaching in the London medical schools, Maclean concludes that 'London presents a picture of mixed aspirations, with many partial plans but few tangible achievements.'

But changes in understanding and attitudes of doctors in training will not be effected by shifts in the academic content alone. Medical students need more opportunities to undertake practical work in community settings alongside other professional course students, including community workers. In the Thamesmead Interdisciplinary Project in south-east London, general practitioner trainees from Guy's hospital work alongside social work and health visitor students on projects in health and social care. A central aim is to help break down rigid professional boundaries where these hinder a proper understanding of personal and social problems and prevent the community-focused intervention which is often needed.

Heller (1978) advocates a radical reorientation of the NHS towards a 'whole community approach' along lines that would be strongly supported by community workers. Two elements in Heller's proposals are of special interest. First, the establishment of a 'community diagnosis' which would study the causes and manifestations of illness and disease in the community; what people do when they are ill; and the range of informal and formal resources for preventing and coping with illness. Heller argues that the traditional individualist approach in medicine should give way to a whole community medicine approach, as represented by the ideas inherent in a community diagnosis. Secondly, in arguing for a redesigned NHS, Heller sees the basic unit as the primary care team. This would be much wider in scope than existing teams and would include social and community workers and welfare rights personnel, as well as the more traditional health service staff.

But Heller recognises along with most community workers that fundamental changes of this order will not take place without a shift in power relationships in the NHS towards a proper representation of the interests of the community as a whole. This will be extremely difficult to achieve. One possible way forward is for community workers to encourage trade unions to become more interested and take action on health service issues. For example, in 1976 the Australian equivalent of the Trades Union Congress mounted a surprisingly successful one-day national strike against government proposals to reduce publicly financed health care.

THE CHURCH AND COMMUNITY WORK

Community work theory and practice has made a marked impact upon the work of the Christian Church here and overseas in the last ten years, though the church's involvement in community work is centuries old. The parish system in the Church of England has contained a tradition of service to a local community, while the church has pioneered many social welfare projects and services which subsequently were taken over by the state. My understanding is that insights and practice methods from community work have been welcomed by a good proportion of laity and clergy, who seek ways for the church to respond more relevantly to social problems in Britain. This kind of interest in community work by the church is even more evident in other countries, particularly Latin America. Conventional theology and theological training have largely failed to meet the need. So, community work theory and practice is finding many sympathisers and even converts in the church, with the process of permeation achieved principally through developments in training and the influence of community workers in and outside the church.

At first sight it is strange that the interest of and involvement in community work of the church in Britain is rarely mentioned in writings on community work. For example, none of the case studies in *Community Work: One* (Jones and Mayo, 1974) nor *Community Work: Two* (Jones and Mayo, 1975) refer to church-based or church-sponsored community work – nor does such work figure in this text. These omissions may be accidental, but my guess is that there is a strongly held view in British community work that Christianity and the church are essentially a conservative, *status quo* force in society and, as such, are inimical to the ideology and aims of the radical movement in community work. 'Community care' is seen as the province of the church, rather than any form of community work that involves protest and conflict. Various examples of church-initiated community care schemes are found in Bayley's (1978) survey for the Volunteer Centre. These schemes are valuable in their own right and sometimes involve controversial forays into the political arena.

Most controversial has been the church's international commitment through the World Council of Churches to provide funds and other support to combat racism and poverty. My impression has always been that there are a surprising number of fellow Christians in secular community work, an impression confirmed by Corrigan's (1975) reference to the church as one major source of community work recruits. These Christian recruits come frequently disillusioned, not with theology but with its expression in institutions. Corrigan observes that for these entrants 'Joining community work is an attempt to take the meaning of Christianity to a modern situation, not in a missionary sense but in trying personally to enact Christian principles'.

Corrigan refers to Christians moving away from the institution of the church to practise community work, but there are an increasing number of examples of the church sponsoring community work that remains part of an expanded notion of the work and responsibility of the church in local areas. Typical of this development is the employment of full-time community workers by one or, more often, a group of churches in large cities as has been the case in Sheffield. The Church of England Children's Society has set up community projects like the one in Bath, where Bob Holman is the community worker. Elsewhere, a church will provide premises and other resources for local community groups, as with the Brighton Methodist Church and its support for the local Community Resources Centre. Predictably these arrangements are not without their problems but they have great potential for further permeation of community work into the church, and vice versa.

Christian community workers employed by churches often experience similar conflicts to those faced by community workers in social services departments. They feel that the nature of their work is misunderstood and that they will be pressurised into work they consider to be quite inappropriate. As with Thomas and Warburton's exogenous workers, they will deliberately underinvolve themselves with agency (church) personnel and not attempt an educational role within the organisation. This effectively reduces further opportunities for permeation of the spirit and practice of community work into those churches. A number of church-based social agencies are employing community workers as part of a remodelling of their function and activities. The Canterbury and Rochester Diocesan Council for Social Responsibility employs several 'community enablers' who have the twin responsibilities of helping local churches to become more aware of community needs and resources, and of becoming involved with local groups and organisations in a traditional community development and community organisation role. This kind of development is a good example of the church, in the form of a social agency, feeling the need to adapt to changing societal conditions, and reaching out to community work for knowledge and methods to enable it to adapt – and, of course, survive as a social agency.

In 1976, the British Council of Churches (BCC) produced a working group report which was rather critical of the church's indifferent performance in realising the potential for community work contained in its human talent and physical premises. The report refers to how 'In the fifties and sixties some clergy, bewildered by the collapse of traditional church patterns in urban areas, were attracted to the theory of community development and readily accepted opportunities to engage in community work. Only a few of these clergy undertook a training programme . . . The resulting projects were often totally dependent upon the personality of the clergyman concerned'.

It was the Community and Race Relations Unit of the British Council of Churches which had provided the most significant support for community work, but two-thirds of the projects supported were not church-sponsored. The traditional authority role of the clergyman together with his too frequent lack of awareness of the social and political processes at work in society were seen as major obstacles to the further permeation of community work insights and methods into the work of the church. But understanding is growing and attitudes changing, partly through the work of community work specialists and agencies within the church. For example, the Home Office's Voluntary Services Unit funded a full-time community work appointment in the BCC, primarily to collect material on existing church-based community work, to educate the clergy in the principles of community work through training of various kinds, and to devise appropriate strategies for promoting community work at several levels. The report noted that the William Temple Foundation was already undertaking an evaluation of community development, which has yet to be published.

Training in community work principles, knowledge and methods for ministers has increased markedly over the past ten years. In basic theological training there are option courses in community work during the fourth or fifth years of training, with some centres such as Manchester specialising in this kind of training. At the post-ordination level, Christian organisations such as the William Temple Foundation and AVEC provide community work training, while some ministers go on secular courses at the National Institute for Social Work and Manchester University. AVEC is a particularly interesting training venture. Set up by the Roman Catholic and Methodist Churches it explores the theory, theology and practice of the non-directive approach to community work in short courses for people with responsibilities for local church and community work generally, or for specialist ministers, or for supporting and training clergy here and overseas. Training in the principles and methods is keenly appreciated by clergy and laity who have long wanted to find ways of putting into practice ideas and aspirations concerning the role of the church in predominantly deprived urban areas. I expect to see a continuing increase in varieties of community work training for Christians because, used selectively, it helps develop a theory and practice for a more socially and politically aware and involved church in the latter part of this century.

Finally, Milson (1975) discusses the permeation of community work in terms of five specific contributions it has made to a fuller understanding of the Christian faith:

(1) *Styles and methods of leadership.* In places, community work has been a challenge to the authoritarian style of leadership traditional in the ministry. The principles and practice of the non-directive approach have compelled many clergy to look again at the traditional methods of organised religion, and to adopt a more participatory approach.
(2) *Awakening local churches to the needs, problems and potentials in the areas they serve.* 'There are neighbourhoods where the local churches have operated for decades, sublimely unaware of the most pressing needs of the people, until these have been discovered by a recently appointed community work team.'
(3) *Change can be effected by co-operative effort.* The collectivism ethic and co-operative practice of community work is in contrast to an overemphasis on individualism in certain sections of the church. This co-operative approach in community work has affected many Christians with something of the force of a fresh revelation.
(4) *Recognising the effect of environmental factors.* Community workers have challenged any simplistic Christian view of deprivation as resulting from individuals' moral culpability. A fuller Christian understanding of deprivation has emerged which does not go to the atheistic extreme of complete environmental determinism. But in assimilating this understanding from community work and other sources, Christians have experienced severe tensions with their faith, particularly those who have wanted to incorporate some elements of Marxism.
(5) *Greater involvement in local community life.* Quite simply, the kind of community involvement inspired by the example of community work activity has enabled Christians to give an expression of their faith which makes them more valuable members of local areas. This involvement may be with the work of a secular group or with a church-based neighbourhood care scheme.

Milson's observations are included because they are further evidence of an extensive and subtle permeation of a major societal institution by the knowledge, values and methods of community work. For reasons mentioned earlier in this section, many clergy and laity welcome and invite this permeation as meeting their needs in contrast to the situation in the health services discussed in the previous section.

CONCLUSION

In this chapter, I have discussed various aspects of the permeation of community work into other disciplines, notably social work and the PSS; medicine and the health services; the Christian ministry and the church. I have suggested that community work is poorly equipped to engage in infiltration of other disciplines because of its own uncertain nature and its marginality in relation to most host professions and employing organisations. Community work has not been institutionalised in Britain, much to the relief of many of its workers.

It would have been equally valid to have discussed the extent to which community work has permeated different disciplines from those considered here, for example education, youth and community work, community arts. A more extensive study would seek answers from research to at least two fundamental questions. First, what are the key characteristics differentiating disciplines that have been permeated by community work compared with those that have remained relatively impermeable? Secondly, what are the principal means by which components of community work become incorporated into other disciplines? In the case of social work and the Christian ministry I argue that they have adopted a welcoming attitude towards community work as offering knowledge and a methodology to help them make a more appropriate response to the task facing them in urban areas particularly. The principal means of the incorporation of knowledge and methods of community work into social work and the Christian ministry has been through training at different levels.

REFERENCES

Arie, T. (1975). 'Community medicine', *New Society* (5 June).

Arnstein, S. (1969). 'A ladder of citizen participation', *Journal of American Institute of Planners*, vol. 35, no. 4.

Association of Community Workers (1975). *Knowledge and Skills for Community Work* (London: ACW).

Bayley, M. (1978). *Community Oriented Systems of Care* (Berkhamsted, Herts: The Volunteer Centre).

British Council of Churches (1976). *Community Work and the Churches* (London: British Council of Churches and the Conference of Missionary Societies in Great Britain and Ireland).

Cockburn, C. (1977). *The Local State* (London: Pluto).

Corrigan, P. (1975). 'Community work and political struggle: the possibilities of working on the contradiction', in P. Leonard (ed.), *The Sociology of Community Action* (Sociological Review Monograph 21, University of Keele).
Faculty of Community Medicine (1977). *Community Medicine and the Community Physician.*
Fraser, D. (1973). *The Evolution of the British Welfare State* (London: Macmillan).
Goldstein, H. (1973). *Social Work Practice: A Unitary Approach* (Columbia, S.C.: University of South Carolina Press).
Gulbenkian Foundation (1968). *Community Work and Social Change – A Report on Training* (London: Longmans).
Gulbenkian Foundation (1973). *Current Issues in Community Work* (London: Routledge).
Ham, C. J. (1977). 'Power, patients and pluralism', in K. Barnard and K. Lee (eds), *Conflicts in the National Heatlh Service* (London: Croom Helm).
Heller, T. (1978). *Restructuring the Health Service* (London: Croom Helm).
Illich, I. (1975). *Medical Nemesis: The Expropriation of Health* (London: Calder & Boyars).
Jones, D. and Mayo, M. (eds) (1974). *Community Work: One* (London: Routledge).
Jones, D. and Mayo, M. (eds) (1975). *Community Work: Two* (London: Routledge).
Leigh, A. (1977). 'Participation in British social services planning', *Community Development Journal*, vol. 12, no. 3.
Maclean, U. (1975). 'Medical sociology in Great Britain', *British Journal of Medical Education*, vol. 9.
Mallaby Report (1967). *Report of the Committee on Staffing of Local Government* (London: HMSO).
Maud Report (1967). *Report of the Committee on Management of Local Government*, vol. 1 (London: HMSO).
Milson, F. (1975). *Community Work and the Christian Faith* (London: Hodder & Stoughton).
Pincus, A. and Minahan, A. (1973). *Social Work Practice: Model and Method* (Itasca, Ill., Peacock).
Robinson, D. and Henry, S. (1977). *Self Help and Health: Mutual Aid for Modern Problems* (London: Robertson).
Seebohm Report (1968). *Report of the Committee on Local Authority and Allied Personal Social Services* (London: HMSO).
Specht, H. (1974). 'The Dilemmas of Community Work in the United Kingdom: A Comment' (Paper given at Annual Conference of the Association of Community Workers).
Tasker, L. and Wunnam, A. (1977). 'The ethos of radical social workers and community workers', *Social Work Today*, vol. 8, no. 23 (15 March).
Thomas, D. N. and Warburton, R. W. (1977). *Community Workers in a Social Services Department: A Case Study* (London: NISW/PSSC).
Todd Report (1968). *Report of the Royal Commission on Medical Education* (London: HMSO).

Chapter 12

THE COMMUNITY WORKER AND THE EMPLOYER

Phil Doran

At the present time in this country community work and community workers exist in the way they do because of government social policies over the past ten years. The rapid expansion of community work has come about because government has accepted current ideas about the delivery of welfare services and has put money (not a lot) into a community-based strategy of welfare provision. Apart from minor exceptions it is the sole provider, directly or indirectly, of community work posts. Such dependence may not be desirable or healthy. But for the present and the foreseeable future, if community work is to continue and to be effective most community workers will have to learn to be effective in a local authority or other public body. This view is one arrived at partly from the community work literature (though literature specifically on employment situations is sparse), and partly from the writer's own experience in community work over sixteen years. This experience has included work in the voluntary sector but has been mainly in the public sector. It has been in local authority (education and chief executive's departments), in the Home Office and in a new town development corporation.

COMMUNITY-BASED SOCIAL POLICY

The authors of the first Gulbenkian report (Gulbenkian Foundation, 1968) on community work training could hardly have expected the dramatic increase in the number of community work posts since their report ten years ago. Their report was one of several documents about that time which set the scene and the pace for the next decade, not only in community work but in the wider field of social policy. Ten years earlier, community work in Britain was generally unknown; the province of isolated practitioners in settlement houses, estates and new towns. The literature was almost wholly from the USA, apart from a few descriptive accounts. Ten years on, a common view is that the renaissance is over. The next ten years will probably see community work stabilise and follow the pattern of similar professions such as teaching, social work and youth leadership. The reasons for these changes are described elsewhere in this book but it will be useful to refer to them here, especially as they have affected the employment opportunities of community workers.

There are several reasons for the take-off of social intervention strategies in the late 1960s. By far the most important reason, in the writer's view, was urban renewal. In the late 1940s and throughout the 1950s, the big cities in this country concentrated their resources and attention on housing programmes in overspill estates. Apart from the new towns there were few attempts at comprehensive developments. In the early and mid-1960s slum clearance and renewal became the task: a process which affected communities more. People were not moving away to find better conditions, they were remaining and their homes were to be knocked down. They wanted and needed to have a say in that process. The experience of the deficiencies of new estates, together with the lessons of renewal in the USA, pointed the way towards a comprehensive approach in the inner cities. Ironically, nearly twenty years on, we are still grappling with the same problem.

Other reasons for an urban review and an increase in social intervention included a recognition that overspecialised and separate welfare services were not helping or even reaching those in most need – especially the 'problem' family. The fear of actual and (more significantly) potential racial violence, following skirmishes in Notting Hill, Liverpool and elsewhere added weight to advocates of change. There was an increasing awareness (reflected in the Maud Report, 1967) that the compartmentalised approach of local government and Whitehall was unsuitable to the task. The size and technical complexity of urban renewal became the dominant feature and drew in the expertise that was available. Thus, several local authorities employed management consultants to tell them how to run their 'business'. A few, such as Liverpool in 1965, even employed community workers. But then, as now, they were not very clear as to what they wanted these people to do.

The government gave a firm push to these developments with area- and community-based initiatives. Influenced by developments in the USA in the early 1960s, government thought it would follow the Ford Foundation Projects and the Model Cities Programme and particularly their emphasis on scientific (albeit social science) evaluation. One view held that the main threats to the nation's social fabric was in the big cities. Social stress, racial tension and unemployment were concentrated there and were also damaging to the politicians, especially Labour politicians. In this way, government sought to have a hand directly in the action, and importantly was seen to be taking action where the need was greatest. Also government thought it could stimulate local authorities to perform better and could also influence directly the results by fiscal and other means. Thus a long line of experiments – Educational Priority Areas (EPA), Community Development Projects (CDP), Inner Areas Studies (IAS), and Comprehensive Community Programmes (CCP) – were all specifically designed and launched by government. These strategies, aimed at the worst areas, were backed up by such measures as the Urban Programme (UP) (Local Government Grants [Social Needs] Act, 1969), Rate Support Grant (RSG) modifications, General Improvements Areas (GIA), Housing Action Areas (HAA) and most recently the partnership arrangements. Generally, government found the big city authorities willing to co-operate in these new programmes. This positive response by local authorities arose because they welcomed any additional resources, needed help and had been trying for some time to get urban renewal regarded as a national, rather than local, problem. The response from government was not all that they wanted, but it was a start. More than ten years on, the £100 million budget for the partnership cities shows that government is still not willing to put enough resources into tackling urban deprivation.

GOVERNMENT SPONSORSHIP OF COMMUNITY WORK

The role of government in area-based initiatives has been described because it is relevant to the development of community work employment over the past ten or more years. Community work in Britain is a government-funded activity. There are, of course, a few exceptions such as trust-funded posts, but these confirm rather than qualify this general statement. Government funding takes a variety of forms. Local authorities are the main employers of community workers, mainly in social services departments, but also in education, housing, planning and even in chief executives' offices. Local authorities directly control these posts. (Though it should be remembered that government, through the RSG, subsidises rate expenditure on average to 60 per cent. It can fine tune the RSG to 'sell' or 'push' particular policies, as in 1978 to enable education authorities to take on more teaching staff.)

Many local authorities community work posts, however, have arisen, particularly in the big cities, through the direct decision of the government. These posts were approved after application by the local authority and then were funded with a 75 per cent grant under the Urban Programme. One can only speculate as to how many local authorities would have created such posts without this carrot. Certainly, without it the expansion of posts would not have been so rapid. The degree of local authority commitment may be gauged better when the funding expires, usually after five years, and the local authorities have to continue the posts at their own expense. However, this situation may not arise because, since 1978, the latest country-wide special funding arrangement, namely the Manpower Services Commission's (MSC) Special Temporary Employment Programme (STEP) also enables community workers to be employed and has the additional advantage that government meets all the staff costs. But it has the disadvantage that MSC decides both the aims and content of the programme.

Voluntary organisations, the other main employers of community workers, are also mainly dependent on public funds, both for their survival as organisations but more importantly here for any programme of community work. This reliance of the voluntary sector on government should not be played down or forgotten. Too often we hear exaggerated claims of the independence of the voluntary sector. The reality is far less reassuring. The Urban Programme and the Inner Cities Partnerships have given many newly formed, neighbourhood-based groups a chance to show their worth, but nearly all of these are wholly dependent on government funds. Even the long-established and well-known voluntary organisations, usually concerned with a broadly defined welfare service, are now dependent on government funds for their programmes of work. Only the big national trusts, such as the Joseph Rowntree Memorial Trust or the Calouste Gulbenkian Foundation can be said to have the means to pursue independent aims. Whether independent aims are traditional or radical is worth consideration because some long-established voluntary organisations appear less imaginative and energetic than many local authority departments.

The conclusion from what has been said above is that over the past ten years the development of community work in this country, and certainly the growth of community work posts, has been directly and mainly possible because government and local authorities have wanted it and have agreed to it. Is government satisfied? Are the employers satisfied? Are the clients satisfied? What do employers want from community workers? The most appropriate employer for community workers is the one whose organisational objective is the same, at least in part, as the community worker's professional objective. However, apart from specialised community work agencies this similarity of objectives is rare. How can the diverging, and sometimes conflicting, objectives of employer and community worker in the state welfare services be accommodated? Part of the answer, if there is to be a long-term future for community work, will require that community workers be more aware of the organisational objectives and structures of their employer. Judging from some of the literature and conferences many community workers are reluctant to undertake this task and will find it a difficult lesson to learn.

THE COMMUNITY WORKERS' IDEOLOGIES, MODELS AND TRAINING

Ideology

Any local government chief officer, perhaps newly appointed, who is asked by his or her committee to report on the benefits, if any, of making several community work appointments in his or her department would find it difficult to make a comprehensive and objective report. One difficulty would be in establishing and then judging the likely effects of community work intervention; a difficulty shared, it has to be admitted, in different degrees, with social work, education and youth work. An added difficulty would be in measuring achievement against the profession's own declared objectives. There is, and perhaps understandably in a new profession, a lack of agreement about objectives among practitioners and writers. In practice, the political ideology of a young community worker will probably matter less than his appreciation of the conditions which have given rise to community work.

These have been conveniently described (Baldock, 1974) as having passed through four historical phases. First the co-ordination of charity (1880–1920); then the quest for a sense of and structure to community in the new estates of the inter and postwar years (1920–1950s); next an emphasis on professionalism because of the use of greater sophistication in analysis and intervention in a wide variety of settings, particularly inner cities throughout the 1960s (and thereby largely abandoning the romantic notions of neighbourhood and community); and finally, in the early 1970s, a de-professionalisation period, with more ideologically explicit claims, where class rather than community was the dominant focus. The duration of this last period is still undetermined though the probability is, particularly with the ending of the CDPs, that it is over and there will be fewer ideological statements and a more professional approach will take over.

There will be some exceptions, of course. It is difficult to see people working harmoniously and therefore effectively in a local authority if they believe their employer is fundamentally against the interests of their clients (though they would not use that word).

The radical community work view would be that because of the capitalist domination of society there is an alliance between capital and the institutions of the state, including the local state, to rule in the interests of the dominant class and against the working class. Someone holding these views fundamentally would want to find ways whereby workers' groups could confront the local ruling class, including the local authority. A local authority employer would do well to check that its community worker sees ways of change other than demolition! Probably, such people would not apply for a local authority job; indeed they would probably not call themselves a community worker as they would believe that it was not a meaningful description. So, who would employ them? One radical writer (Stevens, 1978) has complained that too few radicals can find work. This is hardly surprising. There are limits to the change an organisation or any social system can tolerate: fundamental challenges to its values, objectives and rules are beyond those limits. Community workers, like everyone else, have to work out how to accommodate their ideologies and the practicalities of change, one of which is acceptance by an employer.

Models

Most community workers are idealists; a good proportion are also romantics (very few are middle-aged and over). But, whether pluralists or structuralists, nearly all would agree on one basic objective: an increase in their clients' influence over (and perhaps control of) the issues and decisions which directly affect them. Within that objective, depending on their ideology and particular interests, they will often see their work falling into one of three categories: community organisation, community development, and community action, of which the first and second could be reasonably undertaken by a local authority.

Community organisation is intervention, usually at the local (not just neighbourhood) level, to improve its welfare services by using the resources in the community. This is done by improving inter-agency efficiency and by obtaining additional resources from outside the community; for example, government grants. Essentially this task requires sound administrative or management skills but exercised without the structure and authority that management enjoys in a formal organisation. This type of community work is most suited to local authority departments with services such as social services and housing. The task is basically one of taking appropriate initiatives in the community and seeing that there is sound organisation to achieve the agreed goal.

In comparison, community development is essentially an educative task. It is intervention to increase people's awareness of the issues and opportunities that surround them. The purpose of community development is not better welfare services or facilities as such,. but a new set of social and political relationships between neighbours, workers and between people, officials and politicians. The need for this new set of relationships arises because too many of our social processes, such as industrialisation, urbanisation and bureaucracisation inhibit the full development of a person and his or her basic humanity. Clearly, this development does not take place in abstract or even (usually) in an academic-type debate but through action to meet some practical need or opportunity. This form of community work is often carried out best in an education department, especially as part of an adult education programme, or in a voluntary education agency such as the Workers' Educational Association (WEA), or possibly in a chief executive's office. The community worker's skills required in community development are those of the educator: a person who can educate – draw out – the potential of individuals and groups whether through such basic topics as housing, employment and safety or through the more creative activities of arts, music, recreation and community care. Whether this approach is non-directive or directive, pluralist or socialist does not matter too much, provided it adheres to the ideals of democracy and humanity.

In contrast, the community action approach is much more determinist; it has the economic, physical and recreational needs of working-class communities as its objective. These needs arise, it is claimed, because of the direct and indirect exploitation of workers by capital and the state. The way to combat this exploitation is to make the working class aware of it, and to ensure that marginal improvements in living and work conditions are not used to divert the working class from its long-term political goal of socialism. It is difficult to escape the jargon and stereotyped vocabulary of this field. On the one hand, it is all too easy to produce a parody of the radical left-wing approach and make it look at best naïve. On the other hand, it is easy to exaggerate the importance and significance of the small-scale improvements in self-help, of service improvements and local democracy which can be tokenism.

The issues the radical approach best suits are those that are a clear travesty of human rights, such as bad housing, poverty and racial discrimination. But given the explosiveness of the issues, and the radicals' analysis of their causes, it is not easy for a community worker with that theoretical stance to work successfully in a local authority. A more independent and committed employer would probably be a trust and perhaps, but only perhaps (because many are not radical organisations), a trade union. Perhaps the best employment home for radical community work would be a political party, because a party's objectives and programme are explicitly political. Politically motivated community workers employed by political parties would be more open, and therefore more honest. Everyone could then recognise their aims. But which party? Apart from ideological and strategic compatability none of the British parties which has the resources would have the commitment. The minority left-wing parties that would have the commitment do not have the resources. This indicates the lack of support for many radicals: they simply have no credible constituency. Ironically, it is the state, the bastion, in the radicals' view, of capital, that keeps them employed usually in universities, colleges and local authorities. At least they should thank the pluralists for their existence!

Training

The training needs of community workers were well outlined by Gulbenkian. Briefly these were a thorough grounding in the social sciences, especially sociology and psychology, and satisfactory opportunities for field training. The model was very similar to that used by other professions such as teachers, social workers and doctors. In practice, community work training provides areas of knowledge rather than skill; skill comes from practice and the amount of practice that can be obtained in a one- or two-year course is very limited and gives no more than an indication of potential. A weakness of community work over the past ten years has been unavoidable overloading with young graduates who are well versed in theory but lacking practice. Any practitioner who is worth listening to should have worked long enough in one job (say, not less than five years) to have had to sort out his or her own mistakes. The difference between what we think ought to happen and what does happen is often less the fault of people or even of their false consciousness – sometimes the theory is inadequate and even wrong.

In practice, the operational skills of community workers are more specific and mundane than writers about community work, and especially the writers on theory, would have us believe. The case histories in this book show this. They all describe action to achieve specific improvements in facilities, services and relationships. The achievements are very much at the margins of life in these communities, which is not to say that they are unimportant either to the persons involved or in their social significance. A comparison with education and teachers may be useful. The aims of education and community work are very similar. Education aims to develop the potential of an individual as a person and as a member of society, through the acquisition of certain skills and values. In reality, children go to school and learn elementary skills and information about the past and present and the world around them. In this country that service is operated, for the vast majority, by the state. Naturally, there is a continuous debate about changes in values, structures and methods. The skills of the teacher, however, are more or less the same whatever the context, values and constituency of the school. Whatever their theoretical position in this debate, effective teachers have to prepare a syllabus which will interest and motivate their students to learn skills both of performance and analysis.

Community workers are in a similar position. As professionals they must have a view about the aim of their work. But at work, their achievements are often far short of their hopes. On any day, as the case histories show, they are likely to be making arrangements for a festival, setting up a housing meeting, advising a committee, explaining the complexities of the welfare services, 'teaching' groups of residents, tenants, workers, mothers or whatever, and a hundred and one similar tasks. The demonstrable results of community work intervention, in effecting social, economic or political change, are usually very modest. Even in the long term the actual gains of community work are usually not dramatic and are subject to all the constraints of time, finance, facilities and interest as the rest of the social, economic and political processes.

THE COMMUNITY WORKER IN A LOCAL AUTHORITY

Too often community workers in local authorities are unaware of how decisions are made and of the relationships necessary to achieve results.

The Planning Process

Community workers like any employee need to have a sound knowledge of the operations of their local authority and to be familiar with recent legislation and reports. Local authority duties and powers have steadily increased since the first Public Health Acts in the middle of the last century. The new cause of public participation has spread from planning (Skeffington), to social services (Seebohm), to education (Taylor), to housing (Tenants' Charter), and consumer protection. But there is still a long way to go. Local authorities are bureaucratic systems. They are vertically organised systems which have to service horizontally organised communities (Warren, 1963). The community worker's job is, first, to sensitise the local authority's vertical systems (departments) to the horizontal needs (the interlocking needs) of the community, and secondly, to strengthen the horizontal systems of the community (tenant groups, welfare groups, interest groups on rights, education, recreation, art, and so forth) so they can negotiate with the power- and resource-holding vertical systems such as local authorities, political parties and industry.

Community workers can make exaggerated claims of success in obtaining improvements in facilities and services because they have not understood how local authorities work. Often a campaign for additional resources to a particular project succeeds, but only in transferring funds from one scheme to another. Sometimes this is right, if needs are wrongly assessed, but often it is one poor area giving way to another. To be effective within the organisation, community workers need to familiarise themselves with the constraints and scope of the planning system, and particularly that of finance. Financial decisions which determine whether any substantial project, campaign, negotiation or submission will succeed were almost certainly made eighteen months earlier, and up to three years earlier for programme decisions. Small changes, however, are possible within a large programme and budget, so many community facility and service projects that are well organised can still be successful. Occasionally, major policy changes do occur, often with a change of party – for example on secondary school organisation, sale of public housing, and redevelopment. Unfortunately, the time taken to implement these policy changes often means that the party introducing the change has lost power before implementation and a lot of staff time has been wasted. Politicians would do well to consider this before promoting schemes which everyone (but them) can predict will not succeed.

Councillors

Often a community worker will avoid councillors, or become too identified with one party or one section of a party. The job of a councillor is to represent his or her electors, to be a director of a major service and to support the corporate (party) position. Each of these roles conflicts in some measure with the others. A community worker will not make a councillor's life easier. The encouragement of participatory democracy by community workers threatens elected members in representational democracy (Tilley, 1975). At best it will give them more work, at worst it will damage their political life. The more enlightened councillors, however, often welcome the opportunity to get and keep in closer touch with their electors. But, whether with officers or members, community workers must establish and maintain their trust and respect, if not always their agreement. He or she will not be able to work effectively in a local authority for any worthwhile period unless he or she achieves this relationship. Many of the CDPs demonstrated this – even of those that operated the full five years, many had long before become ineffective in the project areas and with the local authority. Some, such as Oldham and Liverpool, in spite of disagreements, were able to keep effective relationships and ensure a continuation of community work and other resources to the local community.

Departments

Community workers in local authorities will adopt specific roles suitable to their departments whether they are in social services, education, planning, chief executive's, housing or recreation. The attraction of community work to a local authority administrator is that it offers the possibility of additional resources to his or her department from within the community. If a good relationship between a local authority department and a community can develop then a net gain in service resources is possible. Briscoe (1976) makes the useful distinction between community work that is service delivery-focused and community work that is resident-focused. The first is aimed at making the services of the department accessible and relevant; at developing a network of services complementary to its own and calling on the community to augment those services. The second type helps residents within an area define their own needs. Naturally, social services departments are more enthusiastic about the former as it gives better public understanding of their work, creates new resources and gives them support in fighting cuts. In contrast, resident-focused approaches often create new demands without additional resources and sometimes threaten the support of councillors when residents challenge the policies and programmes of the local authority.

Social services departments, which see themselves as having a broad responsiblity towards actual and potential clients and also areas and groups with special needs, generally are much better placed to accommodate both categories of community work. But frustration arises in departments which have a narrow view of their responsibilities and/or have grossly inadequate resources. Those departments also want their community workers to undertake only service-focused community work. They also often have vague job descriptions which cause confusion, resentment and conflict. To alleviate this problem the Association of Community Workers (1973) drew up their own model guidelines for the appointment of community workers. But the persistent vagueness of many recent job advertisements and job descriptions show that the advice has not been heeded.

Where a community worker is well integrated into a local authority service department and is engaged on an approved programme of service-focused community work he or she can become a crucial member of staff, directly contributing to the work of the department and probably also attracting good publicity. For example, volunteers operating a service, providing a facility or restoring an amenity will always attract press attention. In contrast, a community worker in a non-service department, whose work is resident-focused, will often be seen simply as creating extra problems for officers and members who are already overworked.

To overcome this problem a community worker needs to gain the support of key people at all levels. The experience of several CDPs, and certainly in Liverpool, showed that if the understanding and support of the chief executive could be won then a community work programme was in a strong position. Further, attachment to the chief executive's or town clerk's office usually means that committee responsibility rests with a powerful policy and finance committee. This has two advantages: first, the most senior councillors are involved including the leader of the council; and secondly, a policy and finance committee rarely cuts its own budgets.

Community workers without the support of senior officers will be treated as outsiders and will not be given important and useful information. They will not be consulted and will not be able to influence decisions, especially planning decisions, either in person or by alerting a community group as to the way plans are developing. Ultimately, decisions will be based on political interests and power, but lack of information may be one of the weaknesses of a community group, and diplomacy has its place in local affairs as well as at international level. The case studies of Roger Else in Chapter 7 and Gerald O'Hagan in Chapter 6 show how important early information can be in securing participation and improvements.

THE COMMUNITY WORKER IN A VOLUNTARY AGENCY

This chapter has considered so far exclusively the role of the community worker in a local authority. This arises from the earlier argument that community work in this country is now principally a government- and local authority-sponsored and dependent activity. This view does not, therefore, dismiss the voluntary sector as being unimportant. Historically that would be incorrect. For example, the records of the London, Liverpool and Manchester and Salford Councils of Social Service in initiating and sustaining community work in the 1950s and early 1960s are without rival, certainly in the public sector. And in terms of understanding and support for the community workers voluntary agencies, such as settlements and councils of social service and others, are better than many local authorities. because they are small and do not have long decision lines, and they can often respond quickly to need. Also, with long traditions and good local standing, they may be accepted more readily than a local authority and therefore become a good base for community work.

This applies even more strongly to the many indigenous neighbourhood and minority interest groups that have become viable through urban programme or similar grants. Many of these local community workers can, with on-the-job training and support, as Huber and

McCartney describe in Chapter 10, achieve the complete trust and backing of the local community. But, although they may be more congenial places to work (though Dudley Savill shows in Chapter 8 that the conflicts of a voluntary agency committee can be quite disruptive) they are not, in the writer's view, usually effective. However good the relationships between a local authority and a voluntary agency (as between the Liverpool education department and the council of social service) the latter is always the outsider.

CONCLUSIONS

Community work in the last ten years has enjoyed unprecedented academic attention and public financial support. It is a fact that the majority of community work appointments are now in the public sector and the majority of those in the voluntary sector are funded by public-sector grants, many of them for fixed terms. These developments have occurred because government approves of them and is prepared to meet the costs. It is possible that there could be alternative arrangements for employing and funding community workers other than through the direct involvement, for each appointment, of the government and the local authorities. For example, a commission, a trust or council could be set up similar to those already established for race relations, the countryside, historic buildings, sport, nature conservancy and many other activities. That way the policy and programme of community work would be determined by the commission with an annual budget funded by the government. Alternatively, community work could be funded and managed in a similar way to universities. But given a typical community work programme and the traditional and delicate balance between central and local government it is difficult to see many compelling reasons for changing the present arrangements.

The disadvantages of the present local authority-managed and government-backed approach are well publicised. The contention is that community work is too dependent on the approval and even favour of local politicians. At national level, a change of government thinking away from community-based strategies would mean an unwillingness to further fund community work and would effectively eliminate it. The same political displeasure could fall upon a commission or trust, but it might be claimed that the existence of such a mediating body would, at least, slow down any policy changes and even distance them from the whims of ministers. A further disadvantage of the current leadership of government and local authorities in community work is that it leads to a lack of variety in styles and methods of community work: the scope in one social services department is very similar to that of any other. There may be some truth in this view, but the diversity among, for example, social service programmes would appear to refute this. Similar accusations about lack of inventiveness are not made, for example, about schools, intermediate treatment or recreation centres. There is a lot of inventiveness, good organisation and diversity in the public sector.

A different criticism of the present balance might be that local authorities cannot tolerate criticism, and especially cannot encourage criticism, of their own policies, programmes and decisions. It is claimed that community workers who advise and support community groups which are critical of local authorities will be suppressed, or disciplined, or sacked. Again, there may be some truth in this claim, but many local authorities have learnt and still are learning to listen and to respond to the community positively. Any mature system, especially a democratic system, must build into itself a self-critical mechanism.

A final disadvantage of public-sector domination of community work, it is said, is that government and local authority departments are large bureaucracies and as such are unable to accommodate easily the unorthodox role of community work. In certain local authorities this may be so, but there is enough experience now to show that this role can be sustained and can work very effectively. But the attitudes of the community worker, as mentioned earlier, are critical: if he or she adopts a professional approach and is committed to finding solutions within the organisation as much as within the community then there is no good reason why he or she should not be effective.

The advantages of community work being within the existing local authority framework are fourfold. First, there are considerable political and diplomatic advantages in local authorities making a formal commitment to community work, and employing staff would be such a commitment. This action alone would be a significant step towards local authorities extending their task of promoting democracy. The growth in postwar years of local authority functions and services has been overweighted in favour of service provision. Local authorities are our main institutions of local democracy, and that function needs to be strengthened further. A commitment to community work and public participation would be worth having. There is a danger of tokenism, but any small start can be so dismissed and it is the responsibility of the democratically committed councillors and officers to ensure that action goes beyond gestures.

Secondly, a community worker within a local authority has considerable scope to persuade the vertically organised system (the bureaucracy) to be better organised to meet the needs of the horizontally organised system (the community). Several ways of accomplishing this are possible; for example, the formation of interdisciplinary teams and area management arrangements. But the community worker also needs to be an information giver and an advocate of the needs of the community.

Thirdly, a community worker within a local authority department, and especially a service department, has an excellent opportunity to help plan the programme of the department so that it meets better the needs of the community. At the same time, he or she is in an equally good position to help integrate the services of the department and the voluntary and self-organised efforts of the community and to identify any gaps in provision that need special attention.

Finally, the catalytic and demonstration effect of the above roles in a local authority can and has paved the way for local authorities to become more flexible, resourceful and creative in their responses to community needs and ideas. In some measure, a community worker can undertake all these tasks from a voluntary organisation or a self-organised group. In certain contexts he or she may well be more successful from such a base; but with more defined aims, methods and skills in influencing the local authority organisation as well as the local community, the balance of effectiveness is increasingly in favour of the local authority community worker.

REFERENCES

Association of Community Workers (1973). *Some Guidelines for the Appointment of a Community Worker* (London: ACW).

Baldock, P. (1974). *Community Work and Social Work* (London: Routledge).

Briscoe, Catherine (1976). 'Community work in social service departments', *Social Work Today*, vol. 7, no. 2 (15 April).

Gulbenkian Foundation (1968). *Community Work and Social Change – A Report on Training* (London: Longmans).

Maud Report (1967). *Report of the Committee on Management of Local Government* (London: HMSO).

Stevens, R. (1978). 'A fourth model of community work?', *Community Development Journal*, vol. 13, no. 2 (April).

Tilley, John (1975). 'Local government councillors and community work', *Community Development Journal*, vol. 10, no. 2 (April).

Warren, R. L. (1963). *The Community in America* (Chicago, Ill.: Rand McNally).

Chapter 13

COMMUNITY WORK: PROFESSION OR SOCIAL MOVEMENT?

Teresa Smith

'There is one overriding contradiction in the community work enterprise', Harry Specht told the Association of Community Workers at its 1974 AGM (Specht, 1975). Community workers' '*must* deal with the question of whether community work is a social movement or a profession'. Some community workers dismiss this debate as sterile: 'Don't agonise – organise' (Radford, 1978). It does not matter whether community work is called a profession, or a semi-profession, or a social movement – let us simply get on with the job. But for others, the debate is clearly vital, for the definition of community work determines the definition of what the job is they have to do and how they set about doing it.

My own view is that the question 'Is community work a profession or a social movement?' is rather less interesting than the question 'What is community work, and where is it going?' We do not get very far in discussing the first before we find that we have slid unawares into the second. It may be that the first question has a symbolic importance, as a useful stand-in, for the second, more difficult, question. Jerry Smith's claim (1978) that 'community work is still unable to face the transparent reality that it is a profession in all essentials' seems to me an example of this symbolic importance – a statement which appears to be about the profession versus social movement argument, but in reality is about the nature of community work as such. But his belief that the result of this confusion has been 'a kind of collective identity crisis which . . . accounts rather more than community work's structural position' for its lack of results, seems to me less clear and more contentious. So the profession versus social movement issue should not blind us to the fact that there are real arguments to be thought out concerning the nature and objectives of community work, which cannot be settled by deciding that it is a profession, or a social movement.

The variety of activities in community work is so great, and the links between action, rationale and strategy so complex, that it is all too easy to accept everything under one bland general heading and ignore real differences. It is important to recognise that different groups may engage in similar activities, yet have different objectives and different descriptions of what they do. And arguments have a tendency to move in circles, so that we find people doing the same thing they were before but for different reasons – the first and last stages of the Coventry Community Development Project are an example (Benington *et al.*, 1975). Community work needs a definition which makes sense of the variety of activities carrying the label, and the differences in thinking that lie behind the activities. We cannot understand what it going on in community work unless we understand the thinking that informs what people do.

Nevertheless, raising the question of profession versus social movement may be a good way to tackle the job of defining community work and where it is going, because it gives us a good indication of people's views on the nature of community work and where the boundaries lie which separate it from other types of work. What is interesting is not simply what people mean by the terms 'profession' and 'social movement', but why they think the question is important in the first place. In this chapter, I want to look at why people think the debate is important, and what is implied by either definition, as a way of clearing the undergrowth. I propose to look first at what Harry Specht said, then to consider the question of profession versus social movement, and to attempt some definitions of these terms, and finally to draw the different strands of the argument together.

Let us start, then, with what Harry Specht said. He made three comments on the British community work scene. First, the feelings of pessimism, frustration, disappointment – the gap between large ambition and small achievement. Community workers are busy organising adventure playgrounds and tenants' associations, yet complain they achieve no really significant redistribution of power or resources. Second, the mistrust of the public sector, both as employer and as a major source of resources and services. Third, the preference for 'interpersonal interaction' over 'structural change'. By this, Specht meant British community workers' preferences for 'becoming engaged with people and problems and getting into action as quickly as possible', for achieving 'a consensus through personal communications', to the neglect of more structural aspects of change, and the technical skills involved such as analysing problems, identifying goals, devising programmes, building and structuring organisations. His main point is that community workers in this country tend to underplay the importance of organising at different levels, not simply the local neighbourhood, and to underrate the potential of the work they do for organising at the local level.

Specht thought that community work in this country possessed many of the elements of a social movement – a strong thrust of feeling supporting a desire for change, and workers who had come into community work from social movements such as the Campaign for Nuclear Disarmament and carried with them the same 'spirit, ideology, intimacy and exhilaration'. Yet, for him, there is no doubt that community work is a profession rather than a social movement. Social movements may deal with larger and weightier issues than professions, may be 'more dramatic, compelling and stirring'; but they are shorter lived and less flexible, and do not have the same capacity to build knowledge and power cumulatively. If social movements are successful, they develop into institutional forms; if they are unsuccessful, they die. The one is characterised by strong discontent, by collective efforts to bring about change; the other by a body of knowledge and skill within a framework of values recognised by society. Only if community work is a profession can it handle its wide range of tasks and objectives. The question for Specht is how to 'achieve the characteristics of a service-oriented profession because that is the only basis on which we can claim to fulfil the functions of society that we claim we have some special ability to carry out'.

Specht in his paper gives us a curiously polarised and incomplete view of community work in this country, when compared, say, with Mayo's (admittedly brief) overview (1974); and his account of the work of the various Community Development Projects seems odd to those working in the CDP. Some British community workers may indeed value consensus and skills of face-to-face communication more highly than they do problem-solving or building organisations, but certainly not all. The Community Development Projects have been conspicuous for their attempts, not always successful, to analyse problems and devise strategies in such a way that the interrelationships between local and national levels have been exposed, and to build community work into local and national organisations such as the trade unions – although this may not be the sort of organisation building that Specht had in mind.

It is also important to recognise that the discussion about profession versus social movement had been under way for some time within community work before Specht's speech. Throughout the end of the 1960s and the early 1970s the Association of Community Workers raised issues of the relationship between community work and social work, and between community work and other professions; of open or closed membership; and of education and exercise (Cox and Derricourt, 1975). To some extent, this was a replay of the same discussion within social work, dating from many years earlier, and the same language and ideas reappear. The community work discussion has been influenced by the question of the relationship between community work and social work. Baldock, for example, has claimed that 'the arrival of social work as an established profession was the prerequisite for the creation of a new community work profession' (1977). This is misleading if he means us to accept the development of social work as the only tradition, rather than one among many traditions, in the growth of community work; and social services departments probably now employ rather fewer community workers than do other local authority departments, although this may depend on one's definition of community worker. But his claim does invite us to look carefully at the influence that developments within social work may have had on the discussion within community work about profession versus social movement.

Although there is still little agreement on whether community work should be considered a profession, there may be rather more agreement now than there was at the time of Specht's speech that to reject knowledge and skills is simplistic and that the concepts of a profession and of professionalisation are more ambiguous and less monolithic than appeared. Alongside phrases like 'the would-be new profession', or 'the sclerosis of professionalisation', and cries for 'deprofessionalisation', common a few years ago (e.g. Cox and Derricourt, 1975; Poppelstone, 1971), we find far more detailed accounts of actual work on the ground. The rhetoric is still there, but with rather more reasoning and facts.

This leads on to my second heading. What is it that has bothered people about the idea that community work is or should aim to be a profession?

I want to argue that there are four main clusters of reasons here. The first is to do with what people understand by a 'profession'. In the classic literature on professions and professionalisation (e.g. Greenwood, 1966), there is a strong emphasis on the exclusive nature of training, a discrete body of skills and knowledge that can and must be taught, that widen the gap and underline the distinction between the 'qualified professional' and the 'unqualified grass roots'; a move towards an association of 'professionals' with a closed membership, which works more for the benefit of the 'professionals' than for the 'clients'.

By contrast, community workers are more interested in breaking down the distinction between 'qualified' and 'unqualified'; questioning whether 'locals' could not do as good a job as the 'professionals', or even better, querying the existence of a 'discrete body of knowledge' or theory to underpin practice, or the value of such knowledge or theory if it were reserved as the prerogative of the professionals rather than put at the service of the locals; emphasising the 'client's' own definition of the situation rather than the judgement of the 'professional'; rejecting notions of training and expertise as they serve to distance the professional from his or her client, transforming him or her from a committed participant into a detached observer: 'If professional status separates a practitioner from his client, if professional training encapsulates an unchangeable body of expertise, if professional qualifications are used to exclude those with fresh knowledge from unconventional backgrounds, community workers in general want none of it' (Jones and Mayo, 1974). The notion of profession is seen as disabling rather than enabling workers as well as clients.

This rather bare version of professionalism can be met by the counterargument that it is applicable first of all only to a particular period of time, and secondly only to one characterisation of the concept. The link between the struggle to characterise community work as a separate entity independent of social work, and community workers' reactions to notions of professionalism, has certainly been strong. It is hard to analyse this without seeming oversimplistic about either community work or social work. Over the last ten years, social workers have strengthened their sense of a professional identity, partly through the creation of large local authority social services departments, giving them a secure organisational base as the core of their work – perhaps for economic as much as for ideological reasons: the squeeze on local authorities' priorities may simply have reinforced one element of the social worker's role and responsibilities at the expense of any other. If casework has broadened, as some would claim, to take in a wider range of functions than ten or twenty years ago, and if social workers now have a better understanding of social and structural determinants of behaviour, it remains nevertheless true that the framework of analysis and of strategy is largely at an individual level and largely dependent on psychological explanations.

The second cluster of reasons is to do with the question of where community workers derive their legitimacy from, or, to paraphrase Rein (1970) in his discussion of social planning and intervention, how community workers resolve the problem of legitimacy and by what authority they justify their intervention in the community.

According to the classic statement on professionalisation, the basis for the professional's authority is his own professional judgement – his own expertise. The professional assesses the client's problem, decides on the strategy, and monitors its effectiveness. The medical analogy of diagnosis and treatment is obvious. Expertise is bound up with a systematic body of knowledge, sanctioned by society. Professional judgement is measured against the professional practice and judgement of professional colleagues. This does not seem to apply to community workers who see themselves mainly accountable to the groups with whom they work, as the labels 'consumer advocates' and 'servants of community groups' imply. Community workers claim to identify far more closely with the interests and perspectives of local people, community groups, than with professional colleagues. (e.g. Thomas and Warburton, 1977) – and, moreover, use this claim to establish their position in relation to more established professionals.

Rein outlines four different sources of authority to justify and legitimatise intervention by those committed to social innovation: expertise, bureaucracy, consumer preference, and professional values. Where does the balance tip for community workers? Leonard (1973) argues that both the growth of bureaucracy inherent in large local authority organisations and the upsurge of community action and community politics affect the professionalisation of social workers in so far as their authority is based on professional values alone. The same would hold for community workers. Professionals base their values on and adopt their role from the values and standards of other professionals, their employing agency, or those with whom or for whom they work – the clients or consumers (Rothman, 1974). Community workers are more likely to be influenced by the needs and perceptions of the community they work with.

The third cluster of reasons is to do with the question of social control. Professions tend to be conservative bodies in relation to change, with professional associations to guard standards and reputations against lapses. This does not prevent individual professionals working for more radical change, but the radical fringe in professions such as planning or law is conspicuous precisely as a radical fringe. Lawyers prepared to operate law centres on behalf of those who are systematically excluded from such services are just one example.

If professionals are expected to carry out 'certain functions valued by society in general' (Parsons, 1954) then we would expect them to work within a largely unchallenged consensus framework of values, and to attempt to modify deviant or abnormal behaviour towards agreed dominant norms. One example often cited of this social-control function of the professions is social work. At a practical level, social workers do in fact spend a large part of their time carrying out statutory duties determined by legislation or their employing authorities' interpretation of legislation. At a more theoretical level, it is argued that the social worker confirms roles as deviant, and denies the collective or structural basis of problems by individualising them; the problem is defined and the client's behaviour reinforced or modified within the worker's own terms (Cannon, 1972). There is a considerable body of literature (some of it rather confused) on the 'myth of client self-determination' in social work (e.g. McDermott, 1975) showing, for example, how the first reception of a client can screen out certain problems or reinforce others.

For some workers, community work offered the way out of this straitjacket of social control, as workers were not constrained by statutory responsibilities and dealt in collective rather than individual solutions. Popplestone (1971) wrote of the 'attractive possibility' that community work seemed to offer 'for mobilising clients in some radical way'. Yet many community workers fear that current conceptions of community work in local and national government, and employment by government departments, preclude any such possibility and constrain them to work within an agreed framework of governmental policy. Proposals for community work in major reports like Seebohm (1968), Skeffington (1969), Gulbenkian (1968, 1973), were largely made in terms of improved communications, both up and down, and better co-ordination of services in areas of social pathology – that is, the aim was seen as a 'better fit' for the needs of such areas as defined by those in authority, rather than any greater say by the people themselves of such areas as to what their needs were or any greater power in defining the services needed. Attempts at greater participation in planning issues have revealed such confusion over policy (e.g. Dennis, 1972), that some, like Dearlove (1974), have concluded that participation is more used as a tool of social control than as a means to a greater share in decision-making by the public.

There is a further fear that community workers are likely to be subjected to pressures of control and public accountability from both government officers and local councillors, if they are employed within large bureaucracies like local authority departments. Some local authorities are notorious – such as Coventry, Kirklees and Sefton (King and Godfrey, 1975) – for their treatment of community workers who fail to toe the line. This is a matter of political control of the professionals rather than social control by the professionals of the clients, but it is linked to the same fear that community workers have of getting too involved in cut-and-dried professional or bureaucratic definitions of their work.

The fourth cluster of reasons leading to a rejection of the idea that community work can be one of the professions is their claim to be non-political. If a profession is a body of knowledge and expertise which the professionals should bring to bear in treating the problems of their clients, then, while they can certainly define what should be the goal or expected end-product of their treatment, they are not expected to make decisions about different and competing goals. These are political decisions; that is, they are about allocating scarce resources to competing goals, not about selecting the appropriate treatment or strategy for a goal which has already been decided. But this formulation is inadequate for community work for a number of reasons. The distinction between ends and means, goals and strategies is not always clear-cut, and the decision between two different strategies is often a political not a technical decision. Indeed, it may be the political structure itself that is the object of community work, since the issues taken up by community workers are often those which are systematically excluded from the agenda in the political process.

I have suggested so far that community workers do not on the whole want to be considered professionals, because of the way professions are characterised. One element in this is community workers' attempts to disentangle themselves from social work, but the argument would apply to other professions. Community workers' drive for a separate identity, and the recognition that skills and knowledge are important, are themselves elements of professionalisation.

This brings me to my third heading. We have some idea of why people have thought that the issue of profession versus social movement is important for community work. Now let us look at what is meant by the terms in the first place. We should think about the notions of profession and professionalism if they do not seem to fit. Let us start by agreeing that 'conventional categories of profession, professionalisation, professional role orientation, etc. are not really explaining what is going on even in occupations like social work' – far less community work (Cox and Derricourt, 1975). Those who do not like the idea of community work as a profession may simply be saddling themselves with an unhelpful set of categories and assumptions. It is always useful to see what happens if you turn an assumption upside down. Let us take one striking example of this – the term 'client' as used in discussions of professionalisation. 'Client' is a deeply ambiguous term. Community workers shun the word 'client', they prefer to talk about 'consumers', 'locals', 'the community', 'clientele', or 'the working class'. 'Client' carries with it connotations of inferiority, of powerlessness in the asymmetrical relationship between 'professional' and 'non-professional': in the literature, a 'profession' has 'clients' who are told what to do, while a 'non-profession' has customers, who know what they want (Greenwood, 1966). Yet in some professions, it is the professional – in theory, at least – who is at the service of the client, and the client who determines what he or she wants and expects to be advised on how to get it – although it may not always work like this in practice. Why should we not think of community work in the same way?

Specht is clear that 'community work as an enterprise is closer to a profession than a social movement'. Yet in the classic definitions of professions, the game of listing 'essential attributes' is a sterile one – for nobody agrees on the lists, and we end up with an argument about 'true professions', 'semi-professions', and non-starters. What in the classic models appear as deviations from the normal model may simply be normal variations. The ambiguous meaning of 'client' and of the 'professional–client' relationship is one example. Johnson (1972) suggests that we should look not at essential attributes but at the variety in the client–practitioner or producer–consumer relationship and the distribution of power. We may have a situation where the producer defines the needs of the consumer and how to meet them, or where the consumer defines his own needs, or where the relationship is mediated by a third party. Johnson suggests that in social work there are elements of all three, with professional definitions of need and provision running alongside client choice and client diversity, and corporate patronage through the increasing bureaucracy of local and national government. If we accept this for community workers we can move away from the old dichotomy of 'Is it a profession or not?' and can at the same time incorporate ideas of client–consumer choice and consumer-based legitimacy alongside the professionalism of accumulating knowledge and skills. Conflict between different sources of legitimacy, and between different types of producer–consumer relationship, becomes neither surprising nor impossible to handle.

Just as the concept of a profession is ambiguous, so is the idea of a social movement. Piven and Cloward (1978), in their analysis of protest movements in the USA, define these by two characteristics. There must be both a change in consciousness – the system loses its validity, large numbers of people suddenly realise it can be challenged, begin to assert rights that imply demands for change, and have a new sense of their capacity to alter their lot. There must also be a change in behaviour – mass strikes, marches and riots, masses of people become defiant, and the defiance is acted out collectively. For Piven and Cloward, it is the collective defiance that characterises a social movement, rather than any collective purposiveness of intent in the defiance and demand for change. Here they part company with other writers for whom a social movement is 'an articulated and organised group' with 'socially shared activities and beliefs directed towards the demand for change in some aspect of the social order' (Gusfield, 1970), or 'a conscious, organised collective attempt to bring about or resist large scale change in the social order by non-institutionalised means' (Wilson, 1973). This, they argue, confuses mass movement with the formalised organisations which tend to emerge on the crest of a movement. Some people in a mass movement may have clear objectives and a clear idea about their means to reach those objectives, and these may form the organised core to a movement – the more formalised organisation round which others come and go, ebb and flow. And movements must, perhaps, develop this more formalised organisation if they are to survive.

Piven and Cloward's distinction between the mass surge, or social currents that make up a social movement, and the more formalised organisations which sometimes emerge out of mass protest, is important if we are to understand the history of such protest, and the relationship between protest and organisation. Yet movements in this country, such as CND in the 1950s and 1960s, and more recently the Anti-Nazi Movement and the feminist movement, do not conform to their model. These developed not so much from a mass surge throwing up a more formal organisation, but from a small core of people with sharply articulated and defined aims who quickly attracted larger numbers of people and groups round them. So we have a loose amalgamation of individuals and groups, brought together by their strong discontent with some element in our social arrangements or social policy, with mixed interests and a hybrid collection of goals, no clear agreement on a precise set of objectives or means to reach them. Protest movements may spawn both pressure groups and professions. Movements like CND produced a pressure group and also produced a number of people who moved into professional politics on the one hand, and various forms of community work and community action on the other (O'Malley, 1977).

What is it about the idea of a protest movement that is attractive to community workers as a label for what they do? Partly, the looseness of the structure, the emphasis on small groups and autonomy rather than a single rigid set of goals and strategies handed down by the hierarchy. Partly, the emphasis on a change of consciousness, in Piven and Cloward's words, being part of a mass of people who collectively begin to realise their own sense of potency, their own capacity to alter their situation, to protest and be defiant; change in consciousness is both an objective for community workers and also part of their own framework of assumptions. With this, a determination to break down the barrier between 'worker' and 'client', or 'producer' and 'consumer', to claim legitimacy from a common work or social situation – the community worker is thus part of the protest movement with which he or she works.

Yet there are difficulties with this conception of community work. One is that it muddles rather than clarifies the very varied objectives and strategies of community work. Much community work is about plugging gaps in the welfare state, or about 'community care' – which has very little to do with protest movements. Another is that it intensifies the problem about leadership. If a community worker is simply one among many members of a protest movement, then why should he or she not stand out as a leader if he or she has skills and knowledge above the others? Yet few community workers would agree that they should do this. It makes nonsense of ideas of acting as an 'enabler', 'advocate' or 'catalyst' – all far more central than 'leadership' in community work thinking.

The distinction between community workers and local people as activists – 'the "natural" community workers of the world' – is highly problematic, as described by Harry Liddell of the Gorbals (Liddell and Bryant, 1974): 'It's only in the last couple of years that I've become aware of the existence of community and social workers in this area or any other area, and what surprised me was to find that they were doing some of the work that I had been doing for some time previously, along with many others in the community.' One way forward is to accept that the community workers' role is to act as professionals at the service of their clients, as Harry Liddell goes on to say: 'But since [then] . . . I've discovered that there's no reason why we shouldn't work together with the same aims in mind so long as they are prepared to respect the wishes of the community and their desires . . . The role of the community worker would be best served by helping a community to develop its own organisations and help it, in a technical way, to advance the kinds of interests it wants to advance. Rather than that the community worker should be a leader.'

My conclusion so far is that there are clear strands in community work which link it with both the professions and with protest movements, and there are problems with either definition. The only possible solution is that we must have it both ways. As Specht pointed out, it is perfectly possible to be a professional and a protester, only you must be clear which hat you are wearing when. But simply to state that community work is both a social movement and a profession solves nothing and tells us nothing: it is far too vague and inconclusive. We have to try to be more precise about what this might mean, and what the relationship might be between them.

I want to suggest that what we see happening in community work is partly a mingling of both sets of ideas, each growing out of and back into the other. Community work can be seen as a profession to which protest movements have made considerable contributions. Many community workers have come from movements such as CND, from a confusion of discontents with which they still identify, but with a clearer sense of the skills they have to exercise and the objectives they wish to reach. Jerry Smith (1978), on the other hand, argues that community work is a 'profession whose task is to contribute towards the creation of a social movement'. By this I take him to mean that community workers possess a body of knowledge and skills which they should put at the service of local communities, with the aim of altering people's sense of their own capacity for defiance and their own ability to organise collectively in order to achieve change.

To draw some of these different strands together, let me go back to a more important question than that of profession versus social movement – what is community work and where is it going. To do this, I shall look briefly at some of the counter arguments to community work most closely linked with the CDP, and confusingly lumped together as Marxist, and take out what seems to me to be the one key, essential thread that runs through all the discussions – the possibility, or relevance, of working and organising at the local level.

Definitions of community work depend on which traditions are remembered. 'Official' or 'establishment' reports such as Seebohm (1968), Skeffington (1969), Gulbenkian (1973), the Central Council for Education and Training in Social Work (1974), set community work largely within a consensus or a pluralist tradition, where goals are relatively clearly defined, although the strategies to meet them may be in dispute, and competing interests may be rationally dealt with. The relationship between state and community is seen largely in terms of concern about increasing intervention by the state in all parts of life and the increasing size of state organisations, and as a result the need to improve the flow of information upwards and downwards and to create a new or more efficient set of political institutions in the middle. Hence the concern with participation schemes of all kinds, with 'tailoring' solutions to fit a local diagnosis, with community councils, neighbourhood forums, and new forms of local representation. On this version, community work is naturally defined as a professional activity, with its own training to develop community work skills and knowledge, and its own proper goals in the way of a service to be provided for its consumers; community workers take their place alongside other professionals such as social workers, planners and teachers.

Others set community work within traditions of collective protest, of conflict rather than consensus, of protest movements like CND, the student movements of the 1960s and the development of community politics in the 1970s. Others look to community work as a radical alternative – whether to professions such as social work or to the existing political structure of local government, or both.

A variety of arguments about the origins and tactics of community work appear with the label of 'Marxist critiques'. None is addressed directly to the question of whether community work is a profession or a social movement. The criticism is a much more basic one as to whether community work is a valid activity at all. Professions are implicitly ignored as being instruments of social control and conservatism rather than change; the possibility that community work might offer any radical alternative on either a professional or a political level is rejected. The argument is that local action and community policies merely cloud the real issues by focusing on local problems; they are divisive because locality competes against locality for scarce resources, and illusory because local people are encouraged to believe that they can effect significant change in the distribution of resources. Participation and community action may have potential for change, may possess 'the outlines of potential counter-institutions' (Mayo, 1975), but on the whole community work has not succeeded in mounting an effective challenge. It is on too small a scale; groups are too isolated, fragmented and competitive; the typical issues in community work, like housing or traffic, are to do with consumption rather than production and so lack effective bargaining power; and it has been far more effective in the hands of the middle class than the working class. The way forward is to abolish community work – to dissolve it into trade union activity or political action, to 'politicise and unionise', by joining forces with the workers and the clients.

The key thread here seems to me to be the question of the relevance of the local level. The definitions of community work which set it within a framework of professions and local government, or the traditions of collective protest, accept the local level as an essential ingredient. According to Specht's version, however, British workers tend to underrate the value of local organising. On the other hand, we have the critiques of community work which not only dismiss local organising as ineffective and irrelevant but also dismiss community work itself as a valid activity. These seem to me inaccurate on several grounds.

First, to deny as an illusion that local people can effect anything called real change is to turn an empirical question into a definitional one – it all depends on what you would define as real change. It is certainly true that the history of attempts at participation over the last few years is littered with examples of people not getting access to decision-making – play streets in Coventry and redevelopment schemes in Sunderland are two well-documented examples (Benington *et al.* 1975; Dennis, 1972). But it is precisely this better sense of the real boundary problems that we need. The real obstacles to change become most apparent when we push at the limits.

Secondly, it should be local people themselves who define what is to be defined as 'change' and what is not. A dustbin collection once a fortnight instead of once a month, or publishing proposed redevelopment schemes in the local newspaper instead of simply filing them in the town hall, may or may not seem big and important changes to the local people concerned. If they do seem important, then that is where we should start. If participation is simply dismissed as a trick, then real possibilities for action, however modest, may be missed.

Thirdly, to argue that local organising is theoretically irrelevant is to ignore the fact that all groupings draw their support from local constituencies – that trade unions no less than political parties, city-wide or nation-wide organisations depend on organising at the local level for their growth and success. The distinction between 'class politics' and 'community politics' is meaningless; as Jerry Smith (1978) rightly points out, politics should recognise the importance of neighbourhood organising.

Fourthly, if one of the objectives is to alter people's sense of what is possible for them to change, then it is the women's movement that stands out as a group which in recent years has driven home the message that work at the local, personal level is political in its choices.

Fifthly, to dismiss the local level is to ignore real differences that exist between different types of community in their ability to generate or sustain collective action. New towns, long-established industrial and working-class communities, decaying inner-city centres, all offer extreme variations in their networks and their patterns of activity. If we ignore this, we cannot begin to understand how to intervene on any level.

The relevance of the local level is the key to lock together the two main strands of this chapter – the question of profession versus social movement, and the characterisation of community work and where it is going. If local organising is both theoretically and practically possible, then it is a proper activity of community work as a profession. This, indeed, was partly suggested by Harry Specht when he proposed that community workers in this country should pay more attention to building organisations; and community organising is one of the hard skills offered by community workers to local action groups (Benington *et al.*, 1975). The professional skill of building organisations must run alongside that shift in consciousness, in people's sense of their power or capacity, which for Piven and Cloward (1977) defines a social movement. Notions of professionalism in the version outlined by Johnson (1972), and of protest movements as analysed by Piven and Coward, are both essential to make sense of what is going on in community work. My definition of community work is a profession offering hard skills and knowledge, which in part has arisen out of and in turn should help to create the conditions for effective protest and pressure. How to do this remains an open question.

BIBLIOGRAPHY

Baldock, P. (1977). 'Why community action? The historical origins of the radical trend in British community work', *Community Development Journal*, vol. 12, no. 2 (April).

Benington, J. (1975). 'The flaw in the pluralist heaven: changing strategies in Coventry CDP', in R. Lees and G. A. N. Smith, (eds), *Action-Research in Community Development* (London: Routledge).

Benington, J. *et al.* (1975). *Coventry CDP Final Report: Part 1: Coventry and Hillfields: Prosperity and the Persistence of Inequality* (Coventry: CDP and Birmingham: the Institute of Local Government Studies).

Cannan, C. (1972). 'Social workers: training and professionalism', in T. Pateman (ed.), *Counter Course* (Harmondsworth: Penguin).

Central Council for Education and Training in Social Work (1974). *The Teaching of Community Work* (London: CCETSW).

Cox, D. J. and Derricourt, N. J. (1975). 'The deprofessionalisation of community work', in D. Jones and M. Mayo, (eds), *Community Work: Two* (London: Routledge).

Dearlove, J. (1974). 'The control of change and the regulation of community work action', in D. Jones and M. Mayo, (eds), *Community Work: One* (London: Routledge).

Dennis, N. (1972). *Public Participation and Planners Blight* (London: Faber).

Greenwood, E. (1966). 'The elements of professionalisation', in H. V. Vollmer and D. L. Mills, (eds), *Professionalisation* (Englewood Cliffs, N.J.: Prentice-Hall).

Gulbenkian Foundation (1968). *Community Work and Social Change – A Report on Training* (London: Longmans).

Gulbenkian Foundation (1973). *Current Issues in Community Work* (London: Routledge).

Gusfield, J. R. (ed.) (1970). *Protest, Reform and Revolt: A Reader in Social Movements* (New York: Wiley).

Johnson, T. J. (1972). *Professions and Power* (London: Macmillan).

Jones, D. and Mayo, M. (eds) (1974). *Community Work: One* (London: Routledge).

King, J. and Godfrey, N. (1975). 'The Sefton experience', *Case Con* (September).

Leonard, P. (1973). 'Professionalisation, community action and the growth of social service bureaucracies', in P. Halmos, (ed.), *Professionalisation and Social Change* (Sociological Review Monograph 20, University of Keele).

Liddell, H. and Bryant, R. (1974). 'A local view of community work', in D. Jones and M. Mayo (eds), *Community Work: One* (London: Routledge).

McDermott, F. E. (ed.) (1975). *Self-Determination in Social Work* (London: Routledge).

Mayo, M. (1974). *Community Development and Urban Deprivation* (London: Bedford Square Press).

Mayo, M. (1975). 'Community development – a radical alternative?', in R. Bailey and M. Brake (eds), *Radical Social Work* (London: Arnold).

O'Malley, J. (1977). *The Politics of Community Action* (Nottingham: Spokesman).

Parsons, T. (1954). *Essays in Sociological Theory* (New York: Free Press). Quoted in Emmett, D. (1966), *Rules, Roles and Relations* (London: Macmillan).

Piven, F. F. and Cloward, R. A. (1978). *Poor People's Movements: Why They Succeed, How They Fail* (New York: Pantheon).

Popplestone, G. (1971). 'The ideology of professional community workers', *British Journal of Social Work*, vol. 1, no. 1.

Radford, J. (1978). 'Don't agonise – organise', in P. Curno (ed.), *Political Issues and Community Work* (London: Routledge).

Rein, M. (1970). 'Social planning: the search for legitimacy', in M. Rein (ed.) *Social Policy: Issues of Choice and Change* (New York: Random House).

Rothman, J. (1974). *Planning and Organising for Social Change* (New York: Columbia University Press).

Seebohm Report (1968). *Report of the Committee on Local Authority and Allied Personal Social Services* (London: HMSO).

Skeffington Report (1969). *People and Planning: Report of the Committee on Public Participation in Panning* (London: HMSO).

Smith, J. (1978). 'Hard lines and soft options: a criticism of some left attitudes to community work', in P. Curno (ed.), *Political Issues and Community Work* (London: Routledge).

Specht, H. (1975). *Community Development in the UK: An Assessment and Recommendation for Change* (London: ACW).

Thomas, D. N. and Warburton, R. W. (1977). *Community Workers in a Social Services Department: A Case Study* (London: NISW/PSSC).

Wilson, J. (1973). *Introduction to Social Movements* (New York: Basic Books).

A CONCLUDING COMMENTARY

We introduced this book with the imagery of Ivor Cutler's bricks and mortar, in order to suggest how community workers link together people and community interests, rather than being of them; like mortar, their structural position is one of interjacence. Readers, having reflected upon the collection of papers, may feel by this point that they wish to reinterpret the imagery: the mortar to represent the practice of community work, the bricks its theory, values and structures.

The essence of mortar is its adhesive quality: it succeeds in sticking bricks together. What connection does one make, of equivalent strength and durability, between the case studies in this book, concerned above all with the 'here-and-now' of planning, strategy-building and organising, and the chapters in Part One which examine the origins, values and theories of community work, or those in Part Three which analyse organisational, professional and developmental choices facing community work? Undoubtedly, it will be hard to feel well disposed towards the book's architects if they do not help to make these connections.

Indeed, there would be an element of deceit involved if the map which had been provided for the reader's intellectual journey was inaccurate, in the sense of being based on poor surveys or false assumptions. We do not believe that it is. The major hypothesis of the book – the boundary role of community work – is enriched and enhanced by the links and continuities as well as the differences, between the chapters. This is not to deny that community work continues to grapple with the problem of relating theory and practice, as well as with trying to narrow the gap between what is said about practice and actual practice, between ideology and application. These are complex questions. They have to do with the kind of language used by community work and how this helps to determine both the parameters and the tone of debate and investigation. They relate, also, to some strong, implicit values which are important for community workers – loyalty to co-workers and to members of community groups is an example. Such values are difficult to locate and practically impossible to measure. Yet who can say they are not important?

We propose to stay with the perplexing question of how to make more meaningful the links between theory and practice in this concluding chapter. It seems to us that both practitioners and trainers, in different professional settings, have demonstrated increased concern about it, a trend which is reflected in the chapters written for this book. We shall discuss how the contributors throw light on this challenging area, and whether they can be seen to anticipate future development, by briefly identifying four themes which seem to us to emerge from the preceding chapters and which relate directly to the book's central hypothesis. This will serve to draw together some key ideas which have been explored. It will also counteract any tendency to offer a concluding commentary as if further questions are not raised about community work by the organisation and content of the chapters. We are aware that there are major issues arising from the chapters which we do not examine.

1. MAKING USE OF THEORY

Community work has been characterised by a marked anti-intellectualism in the past. Such an attitude is likely to diminish more out of an awareness of the needs of the field than from any sudden conversion to benefits obtainable from academic learning. This, after all, is the context of the search for new forms of support and training referred to in Chapter 1 by Peter Baldock. Equally significant is the growth of awareness among community workers of the tension in their endeavours between total involvement in practice and macro analysis. The former is the action trap referred to by Geoff Poulton in Chapter 5, full-time workers being encircled into local commitment which becomes totally demanding – until such time as theory develops hand-in-hand with practice: 'After a relatively long period of action commitment with people on the estate, during which time there was increasing reflection on the action by all concerned, the team began to be more objective and developed theory related to the work.'

Community workers' interest, on the other hand, in macro analysis of social problems seems to derive from two sources. Primarily it is a response to a growth in awareness of how many of the issues and problems being tackled by community workers and community groups at local level are caused by forces, pressures and policies outside local areas. This line of thought received a major impetus through the publications of the CDP and has obtained a firm grip on the thinking of community workers (though not necessarily on their action). It has been carried forward too by attempts to form borough, regional and national federations of like-minded community groups in order to influence the sources of particular polities.

Secondly, macro analysis may indicate a change of mood within community work about both the likely achievements to be gained by using community work methods and how community work might collaborate more effectively with other disciplines and methods of intervention. We return to this point later. If we are correct in identifying such a change it undoubtedly signifies an acceptance of the need to adopt a more reflective approach: how much can one expect from community work? What is it trying to achieve? What do we need to know in order to make it more effective as a method of intervention and a means of organising? Where should limited research and evaluation resources be concentrated? Lovett has argued that reflection upon action is essential for the growth of community action in working-class neighbourhoods 'otherwise change will not occur except in a minimal fashion with new decentralised administrative arrangements for meeting the social needs of local neighbourhoods' (1975, p. 152).

It is possible to identify two caveats among community workers to current interest in theory, one familiar the other anomalous. First, there is the need for proximity of theory to practice, allied with suspicion of theory which comes too close to scientific detachment. Community workers would sympathise with Berger's confession of rarely being able to sustain an attitude of permanent disengagement even though he recognises the importance of such an attitude being assumed temporarily for purposes of scientific understanding: 'Over and over again I find myself propelled out of detachment by the moral urgencies of the historical situation' (1974, p. 246). Resistance to becoming drawn into over-abstract theorising and a wish to avoid feeling imprisoned by the demands of scientific method may be two important conditions which determine how workers move between different disciplines, and which parts of theory and research they pick and choose to structure their own activities.

Secondly, there appears to be a line of thought which holds that the development of theory must be based on community practice *in Britain*. There is especially an instinctive hostility towards importation and reworking of American theory at the present time (at the same time that such theory continues to be drawn upon). There are few signs of substantial attempts being made to compare developments and theories of community work and related activities in European countries. The interest being shown by community workers in French *animation*, especially by those involved in community arts, amounts so far to little more than curiosity. In the insistence on drawing predominantly on British experience perhaps we can see exemplified the practical requirements of an external occupation role as it casts around for a varied and eclectic theoretical (and value) base. It also underlines the concern in community work identified in the Introduction, with 'keeping one's distance', a fear of being contaminated or sucked in by established professions and agencies, or more developed theories.

It is to be hoped, in this instance, that it does not lead to insularity or ethnocentrism.

The chapters we have collected point as much to the need for community workers to use theory properly as to the importance of developing theory itself. Theory which cannot be utilised as an *aide-mémoire*, a guide to practice, is viewed unfavourably. Grand theory commands little attention. Interest focuses on the construction of relevant, applicable middle-range theories.

2. QUESTIONING MYTHS

There is a striking optimism in Gerald O'Hagan's assessment in Chapter 6 of his work undertaken from Camden Social Services Department. The statutory social services, after all, is probably the setting which has attracted most criticism from community workers (partly because it is a major employer), and we are aware that workers in similar settings could provide contrasting experiences to that given by O'Hagan. However, we do not draw attention to this case study in order to argue about work settings but rather because we think that it is illustrative of *a greater willingness by community workers – across a range of settings – to be more open and honest about their work*. There exists sufficient confidence in the method of intervention itself to make this possible, a reflection perhaps of community work's growth as a profession referred to by several of the contributors.

Such a shift in attitude is welcome because it can prevent community work travelling down the blind alley of stereotyping organisational and employment conditions, as when it is said that working in the voluntary sector is preferable to the statutory but falls short of the ideal of being employed by a community group or groups. There exists no hard evidence to bear out such wishful thinking. Values and ideologies will rightly continue to influence workers' pre-dispositions towards work settings, and their assessment of them. What has to be avoided is the situation where investigation and analysis of the employment locations of community workers comes to a halt. Choices about where best to locate community work need to be based on more than value preference and ideology. They need to be clearly linked to empirical evidence, closely and fairly analysed, not upon pre-judgement, hearsay or caricature. In that community workers are prepared and motivated to open up their experiences for examination in this way, one can be sanguine about the future effectiveness of their work. The first step in that direction is for workers to engage in rigorous analysis of the costs and benefits of their own employment settings and how these affect their practice.

A development which is closely allied to the quality of openness we have identified is that of *increased intellectual rigour or toughness* on the part of community work. This is a controversial area. It touches again on the element of mistrust of abstract ideas and academic inquiry, a fear by community workers of becoming caught in a 'deskilling' process. How can the primary concern of community work to communicate with groups of people in humane and uncomplicated ways be reconciled with an awareness of the need to understand and communicate complex ideas and evolve meaningful theoretical frameworks? What safeguards can there be for a craft or occupation whose essence demands that it always retains the capacity to respond at the level of basic needs to people who experience those needs, and not become seduced by sophisticated arguments and ideas? Such expressions of hesitation about improving the intellectual standing of community work are understandable. Yet they should not be allowed to shackle the ability of community work to stand up to the demands and criticisms of the social sciences. The critical remarks made by Halmos (1978, pp. 81–97) about community work reflect an awareness, by a sympathetic commentator, of loose thinking and conceptual underdevelopment in community work.

Halmos was also aware of the third feature of questioning myths to which we wish to refer, *the dangers associated with reproducing dogma*. Again we suggest that a change in attitude can be discerned here, no doubt associated with the virtual disappearance of early missionary aspirations held for community work. Ambitious statements about 'changing the world' through community work rarely emanate from community workers or activists nowadays. Disappearing too are crude oversimplifications, such as that community work is concerned with collective action and not with caring for the individual, as if the two were mutually exclusive. Increased recognition is also being given to the need to create practice theories which fit particular socio-economic contexts; how rural areas, to take an obvious example, require different strategies by workers to urban ones.

It may be important for community workers to take an active part in helping to de-label community work, and thereby to deny critics easy opportunities of misunderstanding the purposes and methods of community work. There are many instances in the preceding chapters which drive home the point that choice of approach or strategy in community work must depend largely on the particular situation and not be legislated for in advance. In Chapter 10, for example, Huber and McCartney explain why the first neighbourhood worker they describe, Tom, adopted the unusual mediator or go-between role sometimes: 'Tom was helpful in encouraging people to work together and to develop housing groups that are representative of the *total* community. This was not easy, but the neutral role he maintained was crucial.' Theory can set out the different roles which are available to community workers. It cannot, and should not, stipulate how and when each of them can be applied.

The question arises of what effect, if any, the process we refer to as questioning myths within community work will have on its boundary position. Will it be drawn closer to other methods of intervention or to particular academic disciplines? Our supposition is that community work needs to be able to make such shifts, to exploit the spaces or gaps which surround it and restrict it, but that it needs to avoid being neutralised or colonised by another method or discipline. It has a function, in brief, which depends upon it remaining an interjacent activity, lying between other components of society. We shall now consider this further.

3. SHARING IDEAS AND INFLUENCES

A position on the margin allows persons located there to look towards the centre, or towards several centres in the case of community work. How community workers engage in this ability to observe from the outside is important. We have suggested that community work is able to pick and choose concepts, theories and research findings from different fields and use them to its advantage, to take hold of them and convert them into tools for itself. There is here a strong element of exploitation which can quickly become one of pilfering, constantly taking knowledge and thinking from elsewhere and rarely giving any in return. Were that to happen, the boundary roles which we have identified would become distorted.

Community work and community workers can be passive recipients of forces which push and pull them in the spaces available, for example, between local groups and state bureaucracies. They can also be active participants in that process, with the capacity both to resist becoming incorporated by the people or employing organisations and to contribute knowledge and experience to them. It is this last point which perhaps requires closer attention. In Chapter 11 Brian Munday records how community work's influence and permeation of related disciplines and services has tended to take place indirectly rather than as a direct result of any missionary zeal by community work. He explains this by community work's lack of confidence about the identity of its own discipline, 'a constant tension for community work has been the need to look inwards and outwards simultaneously'. Our concern builds upon this idea by suggesting that such a situation can only be seen as a temporary characteristic of community work. Being open to new ideas, methods of practice and other influences cannot remain a one-way process.

Several of the contributors have referred to the significance of both the women's movement and the Labour movement for community work. To what extent does the significance work in the opposite direction? At the practice level, to pursue the second example, community workers try to build links with trade unions and trades councils. What understanding of community work do they communicate in doing this work, as opposed to exploring shared ideologies and tangible opportunities to make links between the workplace and the community? What perception of community work do local trade union organisers have? An activity which is based on the margins cannot allow itself to be placed in a wholly reactive position, responding to events and opportunities, pressures and influences as they arise. It has to be seen to be pro-active, a form of action which has significant values and practice experience which it is committed to sharing with related disciplines and activities. Often this can take the form of sharing experiences and ideas with other groupings and organisations in a creative and innovatory way. Building alliances absorbs a considerable proportion of a worker's time. It is important that it be done on the basis of frank and full exchanges rather than purely instrumentally.

If the position on the boundary does not imply a passive other-regarding stance for community work, nor should it connote insignificance for community work. The two ideas are closely linked, for they both assume a commitment on the part of community work to taking more initiative with other organisations, disciplines and activities than it has done to date. A readiness to promote ideas and influences springing from within community work needs to accompany community work's proven capacity to remain open to and absorb new ideas and influences. Unless both of these happen, community work will condemn itself to a position where it languishes on the boundary of other occupations, including community groups, rather than operating from there in a robust and challenging fashion. This suggests again the importance of maintaining creative tension between the 'in' and 'out' aspects of the community work role – the creativity and freedom available by remaining on the boundary, the influence and resilience it might obtain by moving closer to the centre.

There is a theme in community work of swimming against the tide, of constantly wishing to hold up for examination accepted norms and policies of society. In suggesting that community work should engage more deliberately with other disciplines and activities in order to realise its ideas and experiences more fully we are aware of the genuine risks of co-option involved. These amount to more than a fear of contamination through contact with powerful professions and agencies. There would be a risk of the essence and style of community work becoming diluted. Such anxieties, however, should not be exaggerated. The accumulated experience of community organising serves as a base for resisting any dilution or absorption taking place as a result of the shift which we have suggested may be desirable.

Furthermore, the idea of the outsider denotes the capacity to excel at listening, to be tuned to what is happening and what is being said in different arenas without fully being a member of them. The community worker is thereby well placed to pick up very quickly on ideas or influences which may undermine community work's effectiveness, and to take countervailing action. In this way the community work role itself provides a safeguard against external encroachments on practice. The meaning of the outsider we draw attention to here overlaps with the idea of the non-conformist. It can be compared to the listening and non-conforming interpretations of the outsider explored by Albert Camus in his novel *L'Etranger*. We are referring to the person who, for reasons of principle or because that is the way he or she is, will always tend to remain external to the mainstream currents of opinion; the entrenched dissenter. We suggest that community work, precisely because of its boundary position, allows for that non-conformist or radical role to be played by community workers and that this provides a strong antidote to any institutional threats to community work arising as a result of initiatives it takes.

4. IDEOLOGY AND ACTIVITY

In offering a hypothesis about community work as an interjacent activity we have made extensive use of the idea of tension or strain, the concern of community work to manage competing demands. There is a need to understand and influence the forces and pressures which push and pull community work (at a societal level) and community workers (at a local level) in the space between local groups and individuals and local and central organisations. It may be important for community work to explore the extent to which the existence of tension is a structural characteristic of community work, in the same way that we have argued for the boundary role of community work being a structural factor that is a function of the very nature of community work itself.

The tension is manifest most clearly in the way that society appears to place high expectations upon community work, while those people involved full-time in doing and thinking about community work are unprepared, in several senses, to conform to the expectations. In Chapter 1, Peter Baldock shows how community work has been used as one response in situations of complication and uncertainty. His example of the new black minorities in Britain illustrates our point well. They 'represent some kind of threat to the narrower prejudices of British society'; government then provides resources through the Urban Programme to encourage a community work response to racism and deprivation in areas with high immigrant populations. A similar broad mandate has been offered to community work by the government's Partnership Programme for the inner cities. For a short time community work received official recognition in Northern Ireland as a way of combating sectarianism and social deprivation (Lovett and Percival, 1978). Large bureaucratic organisations continue to search for meaningful forms of participation, and they turn to community work for help. The liberal and uncritical use of the word 'community' (community medicine, community schools, community social work, and so on) remarked upon by John Benington (1974) implies a similar belief that somehow community work in its broadest sense holds panaceas.

The effect on community work of these kinds of expectations is to reinforce the tendency, identified in the Introduction, for energies and resources to be diverted from the task of building up community work as 'a distinctive method of intervention with well-articulated proposals about values, theories, training and expertise'. In this sense, high expectations are certainly unhelpful for community work. It means, for example, that apprenticeship training experiments for indigenous workers are not begun. It means, more generally, that the primacy of community work's commitment to others makes it hard for community work to resist the expectations of society, especially when these come in the form of enticements. Thus the continued drive for action is fuelled, and community work lacks the time and effort to move away from its 'ragged and changing ideology'. It becomes a victim of social change efforts rather than a major participant in its own right.

A preference to refrain from developing a uniform occupational position does not imply that community work is in a position to be complacent about clarifying its values and ideologies. John Erlich writes of American community work that, 'In order to support and sustain their organising efforts, many organisers have come increasingly to the conclusion that a person's willingness to put in long, hard hours is more important than the purity or consistency of his or her ideological rhetoric. Cool commitment is valued above impatient militance' (1977, p. 154). The sentiment is understandable, yet taken to the extreme it risks encouraging even further a situation of activity for activity's sake within community work, thereby denying the existence of the tension which is a consequence of community work's boundary role.

Working with that tension, and being part of an interjacent activity is evidently uncomfortable. Being a marginal person, and sometimes an intermediary, can be oppressive for the community worker. Yet, 'that is what he *is* and what he *has* to be in order to be an effective change-agent within a pluralist community environment of competing interests'.

In so far as community workers do experience Tillich's 'unrest, insecurity, and inner limitation of existence', they may be fulfilling the functions of community work which serve to maintain the centrality of its essential ingredient: bringing people together and helping them to create and maintain effective organisations and strategies.

REFERENCES

Benington, J. (1974). 'Strategies for change at the local level: some reflections', in D. Jones and M. Mayo (eds), *Community Work: One* (London: Routledge).

Berger, P. L. (1974). *Pyramids of Sacrifice* (Harmondsworth: Penguin).

Camus, A. (1942). *L'Etranger* (Paris: Gallimard). Translated as *The Outsider* (London: Penguin, 1969).

Erlich, J. (1977). 'Organising for change', in *Tactics and Techniques of Community Practice* (Itasca, Ill.: Peacock).

Halmos, P. (1978). *The Personal and the Political: Social Work and Political Action* (London: Hutchinson).

Lovett, T. (1975). *Adult Education, Community Development and the Working Class* (London: Ward Lock Education).

Lovett, T. and Percical, R. (1978). 'Politics, conflict and community action', in P. Curno (ed.), *Political Issues in Community Work* (London: Routledge).

Tillich, P. (1967). *On the Boundary* (London: Collins).

POSTWORD

Each possibility that I have discussed, however, I have discussed in its relationship to another possibility – the way they are opposed, the way they can be correlated. This is the dialectic of existence; each of life's possibilities drives of its own accord to a boundary and beyond the boundary where it meets that which limits it. The man who stands on many boundaries experiences the unrest, insecurity, and inner limitation of existence in many forms. He knows the impossibility of attaining serenity, security, and perfection. This holds true in life as well as in thought, and may explain why the experiences and ideas which I have recounted are rather fragmentary and tentative. My desire to give definitive form to these thoughts has once again been frustrated by my boundary-fate. (Paul Tillich, *On the Boundary*, 1967)

INDEX

Printed in the United States
by Baker & Taylor Publisher Services